To my dear friend, EMDB, whose journey and spirit not only inspired the pages of this book but also profoundly touched my heart. As the living embodiment of the lessons in this narrative, your strength and resilience have taught me more than words can convey. You are not just a chapter, but the very soul of this work. Thank you for being my muse and my friend.

-J

CONTENTS

INTRODUCTION

In a world where health and well-being have become centerpieces of daily conversation, there still remain conditions shrouded in misconceptions and stereotypes. Gout is one such ailment, often dubbed the "Rich Man's Disease", but the reality runs far deeper than opulent feasts and lavish lifestyles. "Deeper than Gout" seeks to unearth the true essence of this ailment, shedding light on the lived experiences of real individuals and the myriad factors that contribute to its onset.

This guide is not just an assembly of medical facts and figures; it's a tapestry woven with personal narratives, firsthand accounts, and genuine emotions. Through case studies, like that of Elliot, a resilient friend who inspired this very work, you will witness the true face of gout - one that transcends socio-economic boundaries and challenges the very heart of prevailing stereotypes.

In these pages, you will not only discover the medical intricacies of gout but also learn about its impact on lives, relationships, and daily routines. By delving deep into the personal struggles, coping mechanisms, and triumphant victories of those battling gout, this guide aims to offer hope, understanding, and a sense of camaraderie.

It's an invitation to see beyond the clichés, to grasp the genuine depth of gout, and to understand that it's about far more

Deeper Than Gout: An Average Guide to the "Rich Man's Disease"

Dear readers,

Any journey can occasionally feel like a lonely route full of doubt and confusion. But it's essential to remember that seeking help is not a sign of defeat; it's an emblem of strength and wisdom. There's a profound strength in recognizing when we need support, guidance, or simply someone to listen to. It takes courage to reach out and say, "I need help." Every person, no matter how self-sufficient, benefits immensely from the collective wisdom and care of others.

Remember, the world is full of individuals, professionals, communities, and support groups eager to lend a helping hand, share their knowledge, or simply be there to listen. Leaning on them doesn't diminish your capabilities; it amplifies them. It allows you to gather insights, gather strength from shared experiences, and move forward with renewed vigor.

So, if you ever find yourself at a crossroads, uncertain or overwhelmed, don't hesitate to reach out. The journey becomes infinitely more manageable, rewarding, and enriching when shared with others.

In the words of an old adage, "A burden shared is a burden halved." So, take that step, seek that guidance, and embrace the helping hands around you. Your journey is valuable, and you never have to walk it alone.

Stay strong, stay hopeful, and always remember: Seeking help is the hallmark of a wise heart and a resilient spirit. Please share this book with your support team for insight and informed care.

I wish you the absolute best... and remember, your condition does not determine your outcome—your WILL and resilience do.

♥ JVL

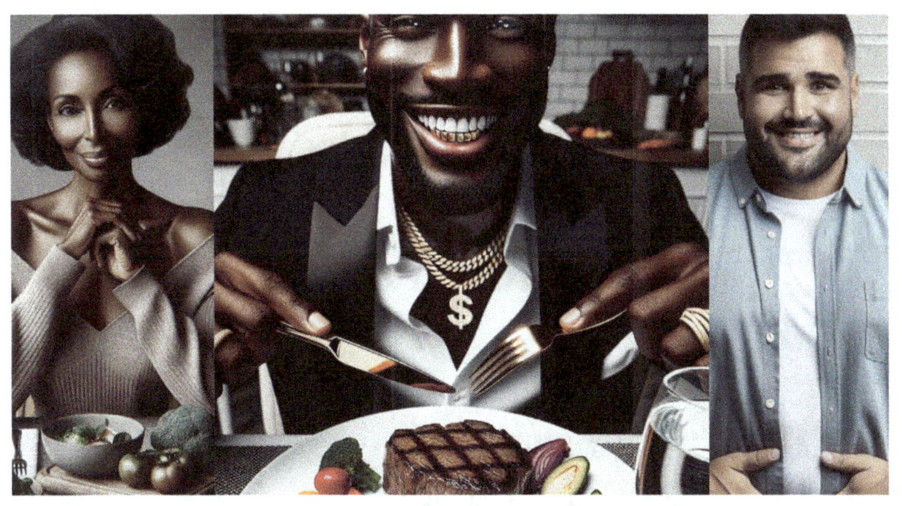

CHAPTER 1 – INTRODUCTION: WHAT IS GOUT?

Gout is a type of arthritis. It happens when uric acid builds up in the blood and causes inflammation in the joints.

ΔΔΔ

Quick read:

Here's a simple breakdown:

- **CAUSE:** Uric acid build-up

Uric acid comes from the breakdown of substances called purines. Purines are in some foods and drinks.

- **Symptoms:**

Sudden and severe joint pain, often in the big toe.

Redness, warmth, and swelling in the affected joint.

- **Factors that increase risk:**

Diet high in purines (like red meat and seafood).

Drinking too much alcohol, especially beer.

Certain medications.

Being overweight.

It's important to see a doctor if you think you have gout. They can help with treatment and advice.

A Deeper Look:

Gout-A Holistic View of the Body's Inner Imbalance

Gout, a painful ailment that predominantly affects the joints, is viewed holistically as a reflection of the body's inner imbalance. This condition is often an indication that the body is seeking harmony and balance. In the US, over 3 million individuals have been diagnosed with gout, making it a prevalent form of arthritis. The cause of gout is linked to an imbalance in the body's metabolic processes, resulting in an accumulation of uric acid in the bloodstream. Over time, these crystals settle in various parts of the body, like joints, tendons, and skin, leading to inflammation and pain.

Apart from the physical agony, gout has implications for the cardiovascular system's well-being if left unchecked.

Gout has a storied past, with it being seen as a sign of affluence centuries ago. This association arose from indulgent lifestyles that included meat and spirits but lacked fruits and vegetables' grounding energies. Gout serves as a reminder of the importance of balance and moderation in all things in the holistic journey of health.

Gout's holistic interpretation emphasizes its interconnectedness with the body's other systems. In traditional practices, it's considered a manifestation of the body's broader struggle with toxins and imbalance.

Uric acid is a byproduct of purine breakdown (a natural substance found in our bodies and certain foods like red meat, organ meat, and some seafood). A balanced body removes excess uric acid through the kidneys. However, when there's an imbalance, uric acid accumulates.

Dietary choices play a significant role in gout's prevalence. Historically, only the affluent had access to rich foods, making gout the "disease of kings." Today, with the democratization of such foods, gout has become more widespread.

Emotional and mental well-being also plays a role in physical ailments. Chronic stress, for instance, can disrupt the body's natural ability to detoxify, exacerbating conditions like gout. A comprehensive approach to health is essential, considering not just the physical but also the emotional and mental aspects.

In holistic healing, gout teaches us the significance of dietary balance, the benefits of natural detoxification, and the importance of emotional well-being. It's a call to action to realign, detoxify, and rejuvenate our entire system.

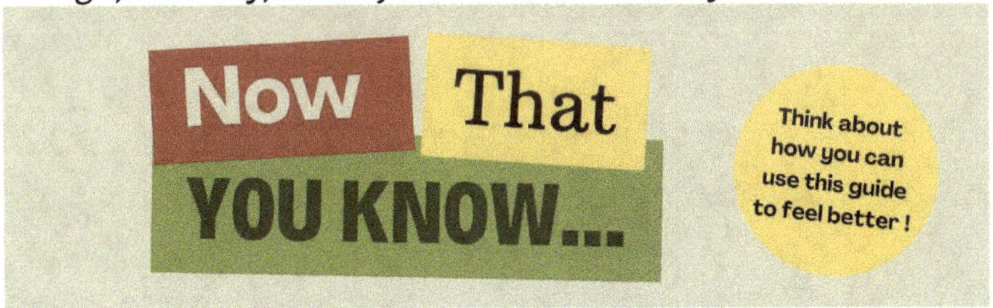

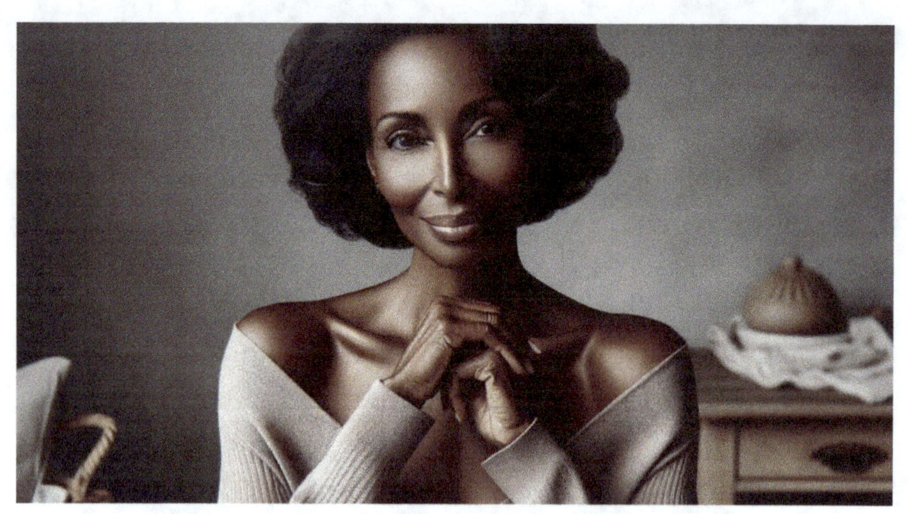

CHAPTER 2 - COMMON MISCONCEPTIONS ABOUT GOUT

ΔΔΔ

Quick read:

Myth: Only Old People Get Gout. **Truth: People of all ages can get gout.**

Myth: Only Men Get Gout. **Truth: Both men and women can get gout. Men are more commonly affected, but women's risk increases after menopause.**

Myth: Drinking Alcohol Causes Gout. **Truth: While alcohol can trigger gout, other factors like diet, genetics, and medications can also play a role.**

Myth: Gout Isn't Serious. **Truth: If not managed, gout can lead to chronic pain and joint damage.**
Myth: Gout Pain Only Afects the Big Toe. **Truth: Gout can affect any joint, though the big toe is a common site.**

Myth: Once the Pain is Gone, the Gout is Gone. **Truth: Gout can come back. It's important to manage it with a doctor's help.**

Remember, understanding the facts about gout can help in its management and prevention. If someone thinks they have gout, they should consult a healthcare professional.

A deeper perspective:

From a holistic perspective, gout is a reminder of the delicate balance our bodies strive to maintain. However, there are several misconceptions about this ailment that can hinder a comprehensive understanding and treatment approach.

Many believe gout to be solely a "rich man's disease" or the "disease of kings." This stems from a history of association with opulent diets filled with meat and wine. While a diet plays a significant role, it's a narrow view to see gout as just a consequence of indulgence. Environmental factors, genetics, stress, and other lifestyle choices can also influence the body's uric acid levels. A holistic view recognizes the multi-faceted origins of gout, encompassing both internal and external factors.

Another misconception is that gout is strictly a physical ailment, isolated to the joints it inflames. Holistically, however, physical manifestations of diseases often have emotional or mental counterparts. For instance, the pain and discomfort of gout can lead to emotional distress or vice versa; chronic stress might contribute to the onset of a gout fare-up. This interconnection highlights the importance of treating the person overall—addressing mental and emotional well-being alongside physical symptoms.

Lastly, there's the notion that gout is purely a result of the body's failure to process uric acid. While this is a primary factor, a holistic approach would suggest that gout might also be a signal from the body indicating broader systemic imbalances. It could be an overloaded detoxification system, a digestive system struggling with certain foods, or even an emotional system burdened by stress.

Gout, when viewed holistically, is more than just inflamed joints or high uric acid levels. It's a call from the body, urging for a return to balance, encompassing diet, environment, emotions, and overall lifestyle.

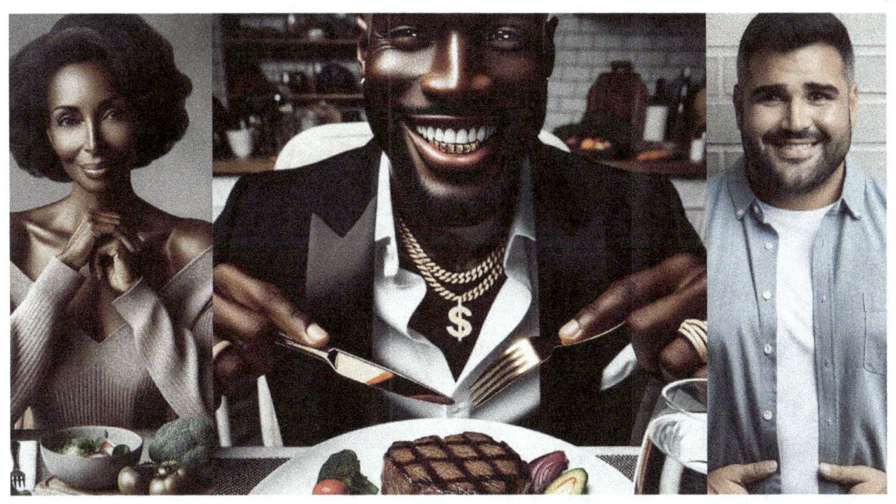

CHAPTER 3 - UNDERSTANDING GOUT

This chapter aims to delve deeper into the scientific aspects of the disease.

△△△

The biochemistry of Uric acid

Uric acid is a waste product formed during the breakdown of purines, which are nitrogen-containing compounds found in cells and food. Normally, uric acid is dissolved in the blood and excreted by the kidneys through urine. However, in cases of gout, the body either produces too much uric acid or fails to excrete it efficiently, leading to its accumulation.

△△△

So... What actually causes Gout?

Overproduction of Uric Acid
- Some people produce too much uric acid naturally.

Under-excretion of Uric Acid
- Kidneys don't remove enough uric acid from the body through urine.

Diet
- Eating foods high in purines like red meats, seafood, and organ meats.
- Drinking sugary drinks and high amounts of alcohol, especially beer.

Medications
- Some medicines can increase uric acid levels. Examples include certain diuretics, aspirin, and anti-rejection drugs.

Other Health Conditions
- Conditions like high blood pressure, diabetes, obesity, and kidney disease can increase the risk.

Genetics
- If family members have gout, you might be more at risk.

Trauma or Surgery
- Sometimes, gout can be triggered after an injury or surgery.

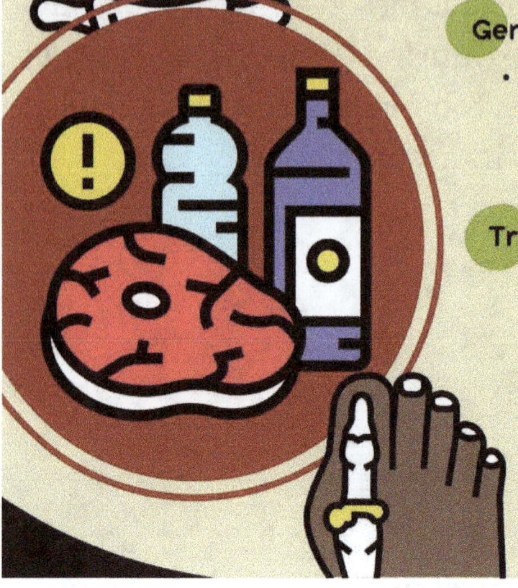

Formation of uric Acid Crystals

When uric acid levels in the blood reach a certain concentration, it starts to form needle-like crystals. These crystals often deposit in joints, triggering the body's immune response and causing inflammation.

This inflammation can lead to intense pain, swelling, and stiffness in the affected joint. This condition is known as gout, and it commonly affects the big toe, but can also occur in other joints such as the ankles, knees, elbows, and wrists. Even though gout can be managed with medication and lifestyle changes, it's important to seek medical attention to prevent long-term damage to the joints. Additionally, maintaining a healthy diet and staying hydrated can also help prevent gout attacks.

The Role of Genetics

Genetic factors can also play a role in gout. Certain genes are associated with higher levels of uric acid, **making some individuals more susceptible to developing gout.**

However, genetics alone are not enough to cause gout. Environmental factors such as diet, lifestyle choices, and medication use also contribute to developing the condition. It is important to note that while genetics may increase the likelihood of developing gout, it does not guarantee it. Additionally, lifestyle modifications and medication can help manage gout symptoms regardless of genetic predisposition. It is important for individuals with a family history of gout to be aware of their increased risk. Taking proactive steps can prevent or manage the condition.

Phases of Gout

1. **Asymptomatic Hyperuricemia:** Elevated uric acid levels without symptoms.
2. **Acute Gout Attack:** Sudden onset of severe pain, often at night.
3. **Interval Gout:** Period between acute attacks with no symptoms.
4. **Chronic Gout:** Frequent attacks and possible joint damage.

Diagnosis and Tests

Diagnosis often involves joint fluid tests to identify uric acid crystals and blood tests to measure uric acid levels. Imaging tests like X-rays may also be used.

Treatment Options

1. Medications: Anti-inflammatory drugs, uric acid reducers.
2. **Dietary Changes:** Low-purine diet.
3. **Lifestyle Changes:** Weight loss, reduced alcohol intake.

We will discuss more about diagnosis and treatment later in this book.

Future Research

Ongoing research aims to better understand the mechanisms

behind uric acid formation and to identify new treatment options.

By understanding the science behind gout, we can better manage the condition and improve the quality of life for those affected.

A deeper perspective:

The scientific perspective provides valuable insights into the biochemistry and genetics of gout. A holistic approach offers a broader understanding of the condition, considering the mind, body, and spirit.

The Energy of Uric Acid

In holistic terms, uric acid can be seen as stagnant energy. When our body's natural flow is disrupted, this energy accumulates, leading to physical symptoms like inflammation and pain.

Crystals as Energy Points

The formation of uric acid crystals can be likened to energy blockages in the body. These blockages trigger an immune response, which in holistic terms can be seen as the body's attempt to restore balance.

Genetics and Biological Karma

From a holistic standpoint, genetic predispositions could be seen as karmic patterns that we inherit. While we may have a genetic tendency, our lifestyle choices can either activate or mitigate these patterns.

Phases as Life Lessons

1. **Asymptomatic Hyperuricemia:** A warning sign to pay attention to our health.
2. **Acute Gout Attack:** A wake-up call to take immediate action.
3. Interval Gout: A period of reflection and adjustment.
4. **Chronic Gout:** An ongoing struggle that requires a holistic approach to manage.

Mind-Body Connection

Emotional stress and mental states can also contribute to gout. Practices like meditation and mindfulness can help manage stress, which in turn can help manage gout symptoms.

Holistic Treatment Options

1. **Natural Remedies:** Herbal teas, essential oils.
2. **Dietary Balance:** Incorporating a variety of foods that are energetically balanced.
3. **Mindfulness Practices:** Yoga, meditation, and other stress-reducing activities.

The Future of Holistic Gout Research

As holistic medicine gains more recognition, future research may focus on integrating holistic practices with conventional treatments for a more comprehensive approach to managing gout.

By embracing a holistic perspective, we can gain a more rounded understanding of gout, empowering us to manage the condition in a way that aligns with our overall well-being.

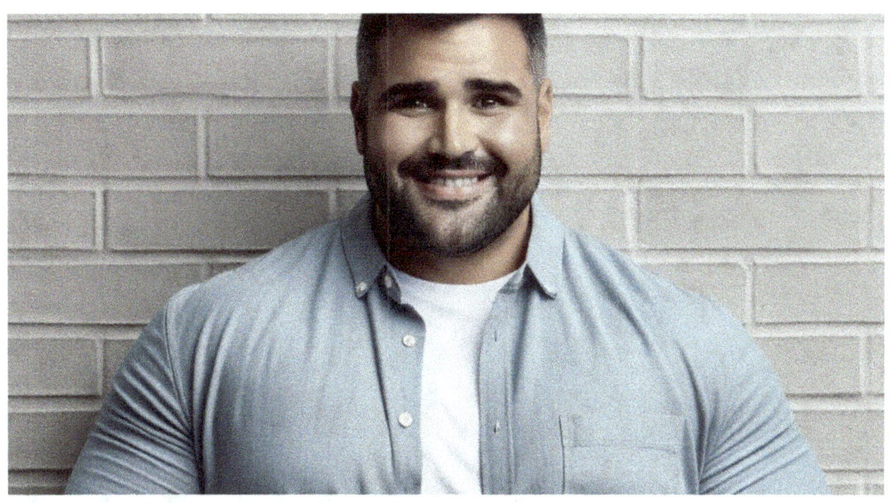

CHAPTER 4 - SYMPTOMS AND DIAGNOSIS

△△△

It's key to see a doctor if someone thinks they have gout. The doctor can give the right advice and treatment.

It's important to recognize the symptoms of gout and get a proper diagnosis. It's key to see a doctor if someone thinks they have gout. The doctor can give the right advice and treatment.

Listed below are the potential causes of gout, which can help individuals prevent and manage the condition. Any individual concerned about their risk factors should consult a doctor.

What are the symptoms of Gout?

01.

Sudden and Severe Joint Pain:
- Typically begins in the big toe, although other joints may be affected.
- Usually more severe at night.

02.

Swelling in Joints:
- The affected joint becomes swollen.
- Stiffness in joints

03.

Redness and Warmth:
- The skin over the joint may appear red and feel warm.

04.

Limited Movement:
- As gout progresses, individuals may lose the ability to move the joint normally.

05.

Pain Duration:
- An attack can last a few days to a few weeks.
- Subsequent attacks may last longer and affect more joints.

A deeper perspective:

From a holistic perspective, the symptoms and diagnosis of gout involve understanding the body as an interconnected system. Each part influences and is influenced by others. Recognizing gout symptoms is not just about identifying physical signs but also about discerning underlying imbalances and triggers.

The most apparent symptom of gout is the sudden, intense pain in a joint, commonly the big toe. This pain, often described as burning or throbbing, is accompanied by swelling, redness, and warmth over the joint. While these symptoms may be localized, holistically, they reflect systemic imbalances. Elevated levels of uric acid in the blood resulting from dietary choices, genetic predispositions, or impaired kidney function lead to the formation of sharp, needle-like uric acid crystals in the joints. The body's immune response to these crystals causes the inflammation and pain characteristic of a gout attack.

Beyond the physical, the holistic approach considers other less tangible symptoms. Emotional and mental stress, for instance, can exacerbate gout. Negative emotions, such as frustration or anger about the condition, can compound stress and intensify symptoms. Thus, emotional well-being is a significant factor in managing and understanding the ailment.

Diagnosing gout from a holistic viewpoint involves not just medical tests but also a comprehensive evaluation of the individual's lifestyle, diet, and emotional health. While blood tests can measure uric acid levels and joint fluid tests can identify uric acid crystals, understanding the broader context is vital. A holistic practitioner may delve deep into an individual's dietary habits, daily routines, emotional triggers, and even spiritual beliefs. This comprehensive assessment can offer clues to potential gout triggers and also provide pathways for more natural, whole-body healing approaches.

In conclusion, while the symptoms of gout may manifest physically, the holistic perspective sees them as part of a broader tapestry of health, encompassing the emotional, mental, and spiritual dimensions of the individual. This integrated understanding can pave the way for a more comprehensive and sustainable approach to managing and alleviating gout.

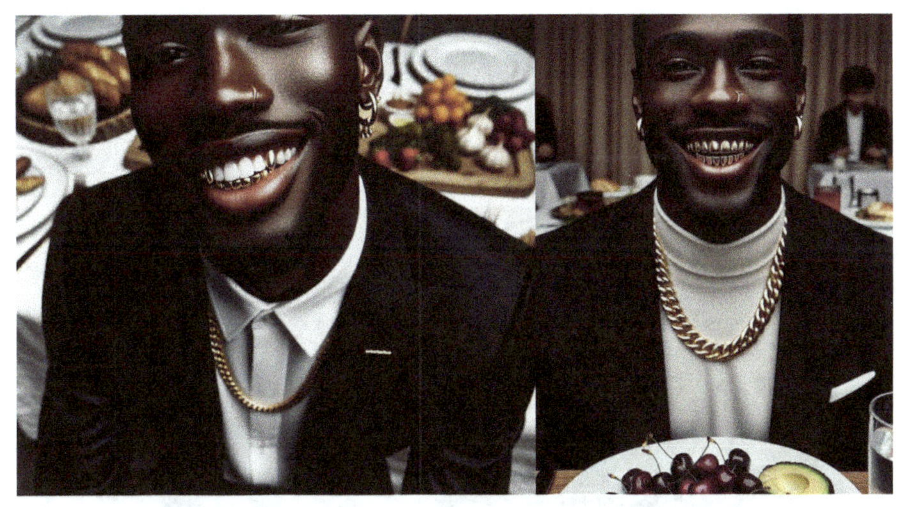

CHAPTER 5 - UNDERSTANDING THE FOUR PHASES OF GOUT

Gout, often termed the "disease of kings," unfolds in a series of stages, each presenting its unique challenges and manifestations.

ΔΔΔ

While it begins quietly, almost imperceptibly, it can escalate to severe and debilitating forms if left unchecked. By understanding the four distinct stages—asymptomatic hyperuricemia, acute gouty arthritis, intercortical gout, and chronic tophaceous gout—we gain insight into the progression of this ailment. This journey, from subtle biochemical changes to overt physical symptoms, underscores the need for early detection, attentive medical care, holistic understanding, and comprehensive management to protect the well-being of those affected.

ΔΔΔ

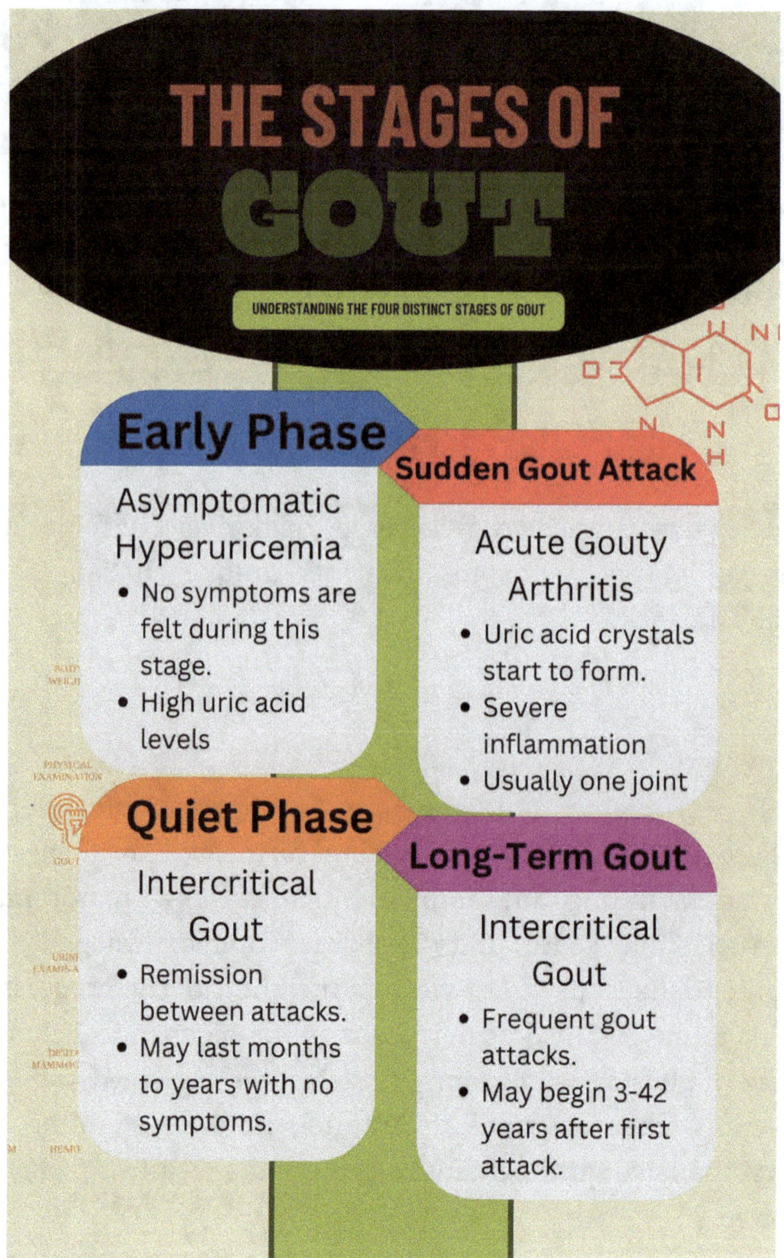
THE STAGES OF
GOUT
UNDERSTANDING THE FOUR DISTINCT STAGES OF GOUT

Early Phase
Asymptomatic Hyperuricemia
• No symptoms are felt during this stage.
• High uric acid levels

Sudden Gout Attack
Acute Gouty Arthritis
• Uric acid crystals start to form.
• Severe inflammation
• Usually one joint

Quiet Phase
Intercritical Gout
• Remission between attacks.
• May last months to years with no symptoms.

Long-Term Gout
Intercritical Gout
• Frequent gout attacks.
• May begin 3-42 years after first attack.

Quick read:

1. Early phase (Asymptomatic Hyperuricemia):

Before any signs of gout appear, your blood might have had high uric acid levels for many years.

Typically, men have over 7 mg/dl and women over 6 mg/dl.

No symptoms are felt during this stage.

2. Sudden gout attack (Acute Gouty Arthritis):

This painful phase usually starts between the ages of 40 to 60.

If it starts before age 30, it might be a special kind of gout.

Things that might start an attack include certain medicines, alcohol (especially beer), trauma, surgery, too much food, and even infections.

Often linked with other conditions like obesity, diabetes, high blood pressure, and heart disease.

Pain usually hits one joint hard, especially the big toe joint. It's very painful, often starting at night.

Uric acid crystals are the main problem in this phase, causing severe inflammation.

Blood tests may show high white cell count, fever, and inflammation markers. X-rays are usually normal.

3. Quiet Period (Intercritical Gout):

After the first painful attack, you might not feel any gout symptoms for months to years.

However, after the first attack, a second one is likely to happen within the next 2 years.

Your joints seem fine during this time.

4. Long-Term Gout (Chronic Tophaceous Gout):

If gout isn't managed, you might enter a phase where it's always there without breaks.

This phase might start 3-42 years after the first attack, usually around 12 years.

Hard lumps, called **tophi**, can form in the joints and other areas. These are clusters of uric acid crystals.

Joints can get damaged over time.

Medicines can help break down and remove these lumps.

In conclusion, understanding the progression of gout is key to its management. If you suspect you have gout or are in one of its phases, it's essential to see a doctor. Taking proactive steps can prevent complications and provide a better quality of life. Remember, you're not alone in this, and help is always available. Stay proactive and seek the care you deserve.

A deeper perspective:

The Four Stages of Gout, from a holistic perspective, can be considered as a roadmap telling what actions should be taken to treat illness and discomfort.

The first stage, (**Asymptomatic Hyperuricemia**) appears before any physical symptoms of gout are obvious. There is an imbalance in the body where the levels of uric acid in the bloodstream increase. This stage might be seen as the body signaling an imbalance reflecting factors like dietary choices, stress, genetic predisposition, and other lifestyle aspects.

Prevention is key at this stage. Integrating a balanced diet, stress-relieving activities like meditation or yoga, and regular check-ups can delay or prevent progression to the next stage.

The second stage is **Acute Gouty Arthritis**. This stage is characterized by sudden, intense pain in one or more joints, often overnight. The body is reacting to uric acid crystals that have formed in joint spaces. Holistically, this can be viewed as a wakeup call that there's a significant systemic imbalance.

Along with medical interventions, natural remedies like cherry juice, dietary changes to reduce purine-rich foods, and practices like acupuncture can be considered. Emotional and psychological support is also vital as the pain can be distressing.

The third stage is **Intercritical Gout**. Between acute attacks, this period is where the sufferer feels no physical symptoms of gout. This doesn't mean the disease has halted; rather, it's silently progressing. Holistically, this period is a grace period, an opportunity for healing and rebalancing.

Continuous holistic care is crucial here. Maintaining a low-purine diet, staying hydrated, managing stress, and engaging in gentle exercises can help in rebalancing the body and preventing further attacks.

Chronic Tophaceous Gout is the fourth stage. This is the most advanced and debilitating stage. Accumulation of large uric acid crystal deposits (tophi) occurs in soft tissues, leading to joint damage. This stage reflects a prolonged imbalance that has affected the physical structure of the body.

Holistic interventions focus on minimizing pain and

discomfort and restoring as much balance as possible. Dietary measures to prevent flare-ups, physical therapy for joint mobility, and emotional and psychological support are essential. This stage is a call for integrated healing, involving physical, emotional, and spiritual dimensions.

Throughout all these stages, it's imperative to remember that gout, like any condition, affects the whole person - body, mind, and spirit. An integrated, holistic approach considers not just the physical symptoms, but also the emotional, mental, and spiritual aspects of the individual.

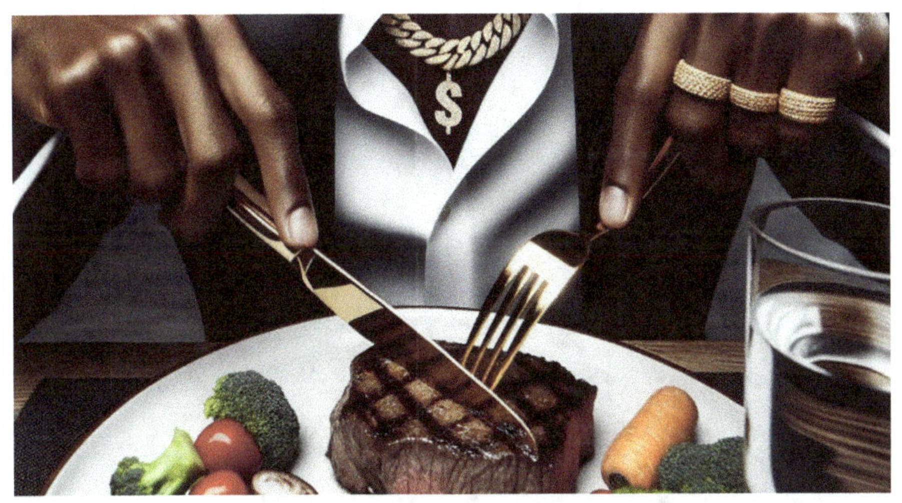

CHAPTER 6 - THE RISK FACTORS OF GOUT

ΔΔΔ

Gout is a complex ailment that emerges from a combination of genetic, environmental, and physiological factors. While anyone can develop gout, several risk factors amplify its onset. Here's an in-depth look at these risk factors.

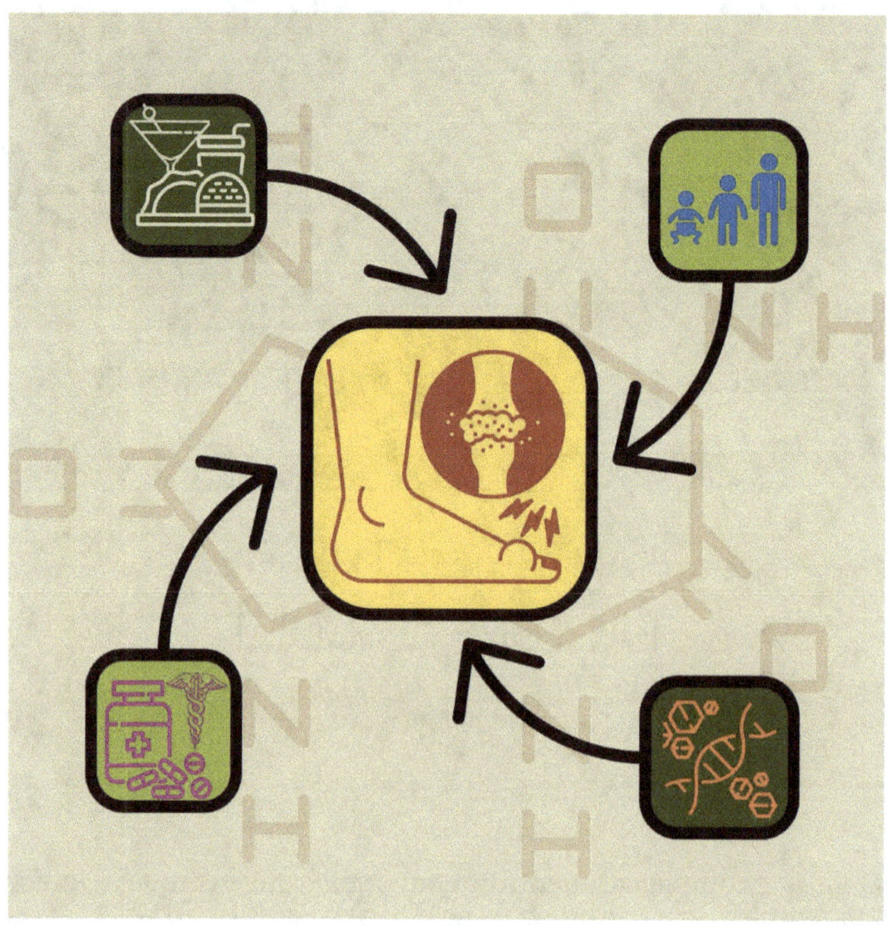

Quick read:

Dietary Habits:

Purine-rich Foods: The connection between diet and gout is closely tied to purines. Foods high in purines, such as red meat (like beef and lamb), certain seafood (like mussels and anchovies), and organ meats (like liver and kidneys), can raise uric acid levels in the blood.

Alcohol Consumption:

Excessive intake of alcohol, particularly beer, can interfere with the removal of uric acid from the body. This accumulation can precipitate a gout attack. Furthermore, sugary drinks, especially those sweetened with high-fructose corn syrup, may increase the risk of developing gout.

Obesity:

Being significantly overweight not only enhances the production of uric acid but also puts a strain on the kidneys. An overburdened kidney struggles to efficiently expel excess uric acid, raising the chances of crystal formation in joints and tissues.

Medical Conditions:

Several medical issues can predispose an individual to gout. Conditions like diabetes, high blood pressure, and metabolic syndrome can alter the body's uric acid levels. Additionally, heart and kidney diseases can affect the body's ability to process and cross out uric acid, increasing gout risk.

Medication and Treatments:

Certain drugs play a role in escalating gout risk. Diuretics, often used to treat hypertension, can reduce the kidney's ability to excrete uric acid. Aspirin can also elevate uric acid levels. Some anti-rejection drugs, given post-organ transplantation, can further exacerbate the risk.

Genetics and Family History:

Genetics plays a significant role in many ailments, including gout. If your parents or grandparents battled gout, your risk is inherently higher. This genetic predisposition underscores the importance of early detection and lifestyle modifications.

Age and Gender Dynamics:

Gout has a marked gender bias. Men, particularly between the ages of 30 and 50, are at heightened risk. While women can also develop gout, their susceptibility significantly increases post-menopause, when the protective effects of estrogen, which aids in uric acid excretion, diminish.

Recent Physical Distress:

Surprisingly, events like surgeries or severe trauma can act as triggers for a gout attack. The exact mechanisms remain under research, but it's essential to track and manage uric acid levels during recovery from such events.

Understanding these risk factors is paramount in adopting a preventive approach. By being aware of the causes and making appropriate lifestyle choices, one can significantly mitigate the risk of developing gout or manage it more effectively if already diagnosed.

<u>A deeper perspective:</u>

Gout, while deeply rooted in our body's biological and biochemical processes, is a condition that finds its origins and aggravators in an interplay of factors, both internal and external. The holistic perspective delves deeper than mere symptoms; it seeks to understand the broader environment and lifestyle influences that come into play. From what we consume to how we live; various aspects mold our vulnerability to gout. This chapter unfolds a comprehensive exploration of these risk factors, anchoring our understanding not just in the physiological but also in the environmental, emotional, and energetic realms.

Dietary Influences:

Central to holistic thought is the ancient adage, "You are what you eat." The food choices we make can significantly impact our health and well-being. Diets abundant in purine-rich foods such as red meat, certain seafood, and organ meats contribute to higher levels of uric acid, a precursor to gout. Moreover, excessive alcohol consumption, especially beer, and indulgence in sugary beverages can upset the body's metabolic balance, fostering an environment conducive to gout attacks. As such, maintaining a balanced diet, rich in anti-inflammatory foods and low in high-purine content, can be a preventive strategy.

The Weight of Obesity:

Carrying excess weight does more than just strain our joints and bones; it has cascading effects on our overall health. Obesity can escalate the body's production of uric acid and simultaneously challenge the kidneys in effectively filtering it out. From a holistic standpoint, the body's energy flow or "chi" can be compromised by obesity, leading to stagnation and imbalance amplifying gout's onset.

Underlying Medical Conditions:

Our body systems are intricately connected, and the malfunction of one can ripple effects across others. Conditions like diabetes, high blood pressure, metabolic syndrome, and heart or kidney diseases not only stand as health challenges on their own but also heighten the risk of gout. Holistically, these conditions signify a break in the body's harmony, requiring a multi-dimensional approach to healing and prevention.

Medications and Their Dual-Edged Sword:

Certain drugs, though beneficial for their primary purposes, can inadvertently raise uric acid levels. Diuretics, specific anti-rejection drugs, and even common aspirins come under this umbrella. While medications are sometimes essential, understanding their broader impacts and seeking natural, complementary therapies can provide a more rounded approach to health.

The Threads of Family and Genetics:
While we are unique beings, our genetic tapestry draws heavily from our ancestors. A family history of gout can predispose individuals to this condition. This genetic inclination is not just about DNA but also about shared lifestyles, habits, and environments that families often have in common.

The Dance of Age and Gender:

Life's natural phases bring about shifts in our body's chemistry and functioning. Men, especially between the ages of 30 to 50, are more susceptible to gout. Women, on the other hand, see their risk rise post-menopause, likely due to the diminishing protective efects of estrogen. Respecting these natural rhythms and adapting our lifestyles can play a role in risk mitigation.

Physical Trauma and Its Ripples:

Our bodies, while resilient, are also sensitive to disruptions. Recent surgeries or physical traumas can sometimes serve as triggers for gout attacks. Such events, beyond their immediate physical impact, can also disturb the body's energetic balance, highlighting the importance of holistic healing and care post any form of trauma.

In conclusion, while the risk factors for gout are multifaceted, the holistic lens ofers a broader, more integrated understanding. By recognizing and addressing these factors, not in isolation but as part of the greater whole, we can embark on a more comprehensive journey towards health, balance, and well-being.

Diving Deeper: Understanding the Graver Implications of Gout

Gout, often dismissed as a fleeting discomfort or an isolated joint concern, can manifest deeper repercussions when left unchecked. What begin as sporadic pain episodes can morph into more chronic and severe health challenges. Recognizing these indicators early on is pivotal, not just for managing gout, but for safeguarding one's overall well-being. Let's delve into these significant health signals linked to gout's progression:

The Alarming Frequency of Attacks:

When gout fare-ups become a recurrent theme, it's a telling sign that the condition isn't under optimal control. These repeated episodes, beyond the immediate pain and discomfort, serve as a harbinger of potential joint deterioration.

The Wear and Tear of Joints:

A long-standing battle with gout, especially when inadequately addressed, can lead to tangible damage within the joints. This erosion compromises the joint's structural integrity, leading to reduced mobility and an impaired quality of life.

The Emergence of Tophi:

These aren't just benign lumps but are crystallized indicators of a deeper problem. Tophi, which are hard nodules of uric acid, often materialize around joints and are emblematic of chronic, unregulated gout. Their presence underscores the urgent need for intervention and more stringent gout management.

The Stone Trail to the Kidneys:

The excess uric acid, the very culprit behind gout, can also journey to the kidneys. Here, it can congregate and form stones, adding another layer of health complication and discomfort.

The Silent Progression to Kidney Disease:

Gout doesn't just stop at forming stones. If left unbridled, it can escalate to a point where it starts to impede the kidneys' functioning, inching one closer to renal disease. The kidneys, essential for filtering out toxins, when compromised, can set off a cascade of health issues.

The Heart Connection:

The heart, our vital life pump, isn't immune to gout's effects. Emerging research has drawn connections between persistent gout and heightened risk for cardiovascular challenges. While the exact pathways are still under investigation, the link accentuates the importance of holistic health vigilance for gout patients.

Gout isn't a condition to be taken lightly. Its tentacles can reach various organs and systems, emphasizing the need for proactive management, comprehensive care, and regular health check-ups.

Gout, while known for its episodic fare-ups, occasionally presents symptoms that go beyond the usual discomfort and pain. These intensified signs are crucial red flags, signifying potential complications or an aggravated state of the condition. Ignoring these symptoms not only prolongs suffering but can lead to lasting damage. Here are some gout symptoms that should set off alarm bells:

Prolonged Intense Pain:

While gout attacks are notoriously painful, if you experience excruciating pain that doesn't show signs of subsiding after the first 24 hours or persists beyond a week, it's essential to consult a healthcare professional.

Multiple Joint Involvement:

Gout commonly targets the big toe. However, if multiple joints are affected simultaneously, especially in the early stages of the disease, it's a sign of a rapid and aggressive form of gout that requires medical attention.

Severe Redness and Warmth:

A fiery red hue and warmth over the affected joint, particularly if a fever goes with it, might indicate an infection or a condition called septic arthritis. This needs urgent medical evaluation.

Presence of Tophi:

If you notice hard lumps under your skin around the joints or other areas like the ears, you're observing tophi. These are accumulations of uric acid crystals and signify chronic gout. They can lead to joint damage and other complications if not addressed.

Reduced Range of Motion:

If your ability to move a joint is severely restricted or if the joint becomes rigid, it might indicate extensive joint damage or developing conditions like osteoarthritis alongside gout.

Persistent Fatigue:

While fatigue isn't a direct symptom of gout, persistent tiredness, especially after a gout attack, should not be overlooked. It could be indicative of related complications or other underlying health issues.

Changes in Urine or Kidney Pain:

Dark, cloudy urine, pain on one side of the lower back, or decreased urine output can hint at kidney stones or kidney disease, often linked to prolonged high uric acid levels.

Rapid Onset of Attacks:

If gout attacks are happening more often and with little to no known triggers, it signifies an escalation of the disease, demanding a reevaluation of your management strategy.

Remember, while gout can be managed with lifestyle adjustments and medications, some symptoms indicate a progression or complication that needs medical intervention. Always prioritize your health and seek guidance when faced with alarming symptoms. The key is to act promptly and avoid potential long-term damage.

It's crucial to manage gout properly. If someone sees these serious indicators, they should see a doctor immediately. Regular check-ups can also help catch and address issues early.

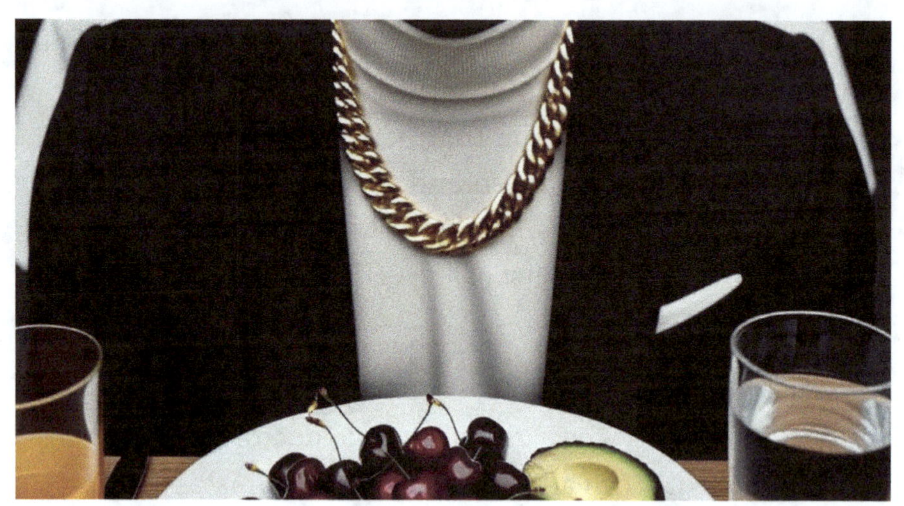

CHAPTER 7 – UNDERSTANDING THE RELATIONSHIP BETWEEN GOUT AND DIET

△△△

Gout is closely intertwined with the foods and drinks we consume. Specific dietary choices can exacerbate or trigger gout symptoms due to the impact they have on uric acid levels in the body. This chapter delves into the dietary factors that influence gout and provides a clearer understanding of what to approach with caution.

Quick read:

Purines and Uric Acid Production

Purines are compounds found naturally in many foods. When digested, they break down to form uric acid. For individuals prone to gout, foods high in purines can lead to increased uric acid levels and crystallization in the joints. Key foods to be cautious of include:

Red Meats and Organ Meats: Foods like beef, lamb, and organ meats such as liver and kidneys have a high purine content.

Certain Seafoods: While seafood has its health benefits, some types, including shrimp, mussels, and certain fish like sardines and mackerel, can contribute to uric acid production.

Alcohol's Impact on Gout

Alcohol, especially beer, affects how the body handles uric acid. It can impede the removal process, leading to increased levels in the bloodstream and potential gout fare-ups.

Sugary Foods and Drinks

High-fructose foods and drinks, including sodas, fruit juices with added sugar, and candies, can elevate uric acid levels, posing a risk for gout attacks.

Vegetables with Purines

Some vegetables, like spinach, asparagus, and cauliflower, contain purines. While their contribution to gout is less than that of meat, it's essential to be aware of them.

Processed Foods and Gout

Many processed foods, from snacks to some meats, might contain ingredients that elevate uric acid levels. Checking ingredient lists and being aware of purine sources can help in making informed food choices.

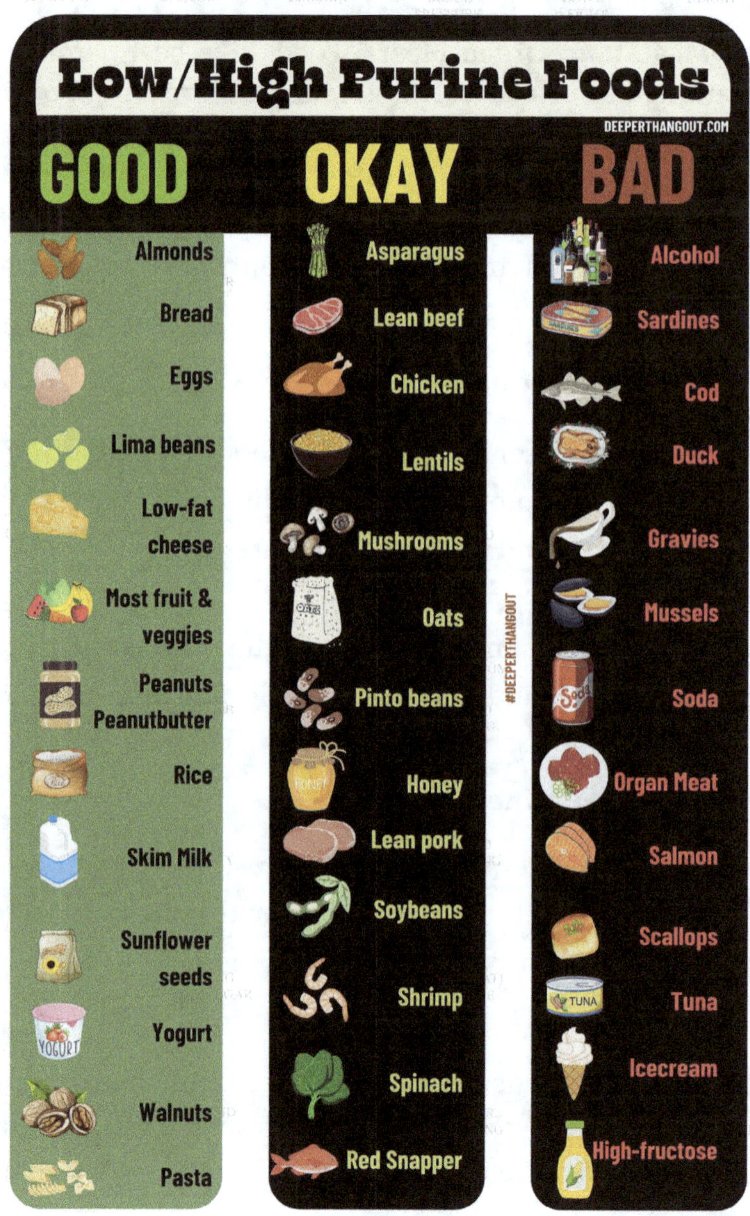

In conclusion, understanding the dietary triggers for gout and being aware of the foods and drinks that impact uric acid levels can support individuals in making choices that support their health and well-being.

Managing Gout Through Holistic and Natural Healing

In the realm of holistic health and natural healing, gout is viewed not merely as a standalone ailment but as a reflection of overall body imbalances. Addressing gout from this perspective means understanding its root causes and employing natural remedies and lifestyle changes to restore balance. This chapter delves into holistic approaches and natural healing methods for managing gout.

1. Dietary Awareness: The Foundation of Balance

Gout fare-ups are closely tied to dietary choices. Consuming high-purine foods such as red meats, organ meats, seafood, certain vegetables, and processed foods can lead to elevated uric acid levels. From a holistic viewpoint, it's essential to nourish the body with whole, natural foods that promote balance:

Alkaline-rich Foods: Leafy greens, celery, cherries, and apples can help neutralize excess acidity in the body, reducing the risk of uric acid buildup.

Hydration: Drinking plenty of water aids in flushing out toxins and excess uric acid from the body.

2. Herbal Allies for Gout Relief

Nature offers an array of herbs that can support the body in managing gout:

Nettle Leaf: Known for its diuretic properties, nettle leaf can help remove uric acid from the body.

Turmeric and Ginger: Both carry anti-inflammatory properties that can alleviate joint pain and inflammation associated with gout.

3. Mind-Body Practices

Stress can exacerbate gout symptoms. Engaging in mind-body practices can provide relief:

Meditation and Deep Breathing: These practices can help in managing stress, reducing inflammation, and promoting overall well-being.

Gentle Movement: Yoga and Tai Chi can improve joint flexibility and reduce stress, benefiting those with gout.

4. External Natural Remedies

Applying natural substances externally can offer relief from gout pain:

Epsom Salt Baths: The magnesium in Epsom salt can relax muscles and reduce inflammation.

Cold Compress: Applying a cold compress to the affected joint can reduce swelling and pain.

5. The Power of Prevention

Prevention is a cornerstone of holistic health. Regular check-ups, understanding one's family history, and being attuned to the body's signals can help prevent severe gout flare-ups.

6. Integrative Approaches

While natural remedies can offer relief, it's essential to understand that severe gout might require a combination of holistic and conventional treatments. It's always advisable to consult with healthcare professionals when considering any treatment plan.

Conclusion

Holistic and natural healing approaches offer a comprehensive way to manage gout, emphasizing the interconnectedness of body, mind, and spirit. By adopting a holistic lifestyle and integrating natural remedies, individuals can navigate their gout journey with resilience and grace.

It's important to note that everyone is different. Some people might be more sensitive to certain foods than others. If someone suspects a specific food is triggering their gout, it's a good idea to discuss it with a doctor or nutritionist. They can help create a diet plan that reduces the risk of gout attacks.

Recommended Dietary Choices for Gout Sufferers

Regarding managing gout, dietary choices play a pivotal role. Here are some food recommendations that can help in reducing the risk of gout fare-ups and promoting overall well-being:

1. Low-Purine Foods:

Foods that are low in purines are less likely to raise uric acid levels in the blood.

Fruits: Cherries are particularly beneficial for gout sufferers due to compounds that might help lower uric acid. Other fruits are also generally safe.

Vegetables: Opt for low-purine vegetables such as bell peppers, carrots, and cucumbers.

Whole Grains: Incorporate grains like oats, brown rice, and quinoa into the diet.

2. Dairy Products:

Benefits: Low-fat dairy products not only provide essential nutrients but also aid in removing uric acid from the body.

Options: Include low-fat yogurt, milk, and cheese in the diet for their potential gout-preventing properties.

3. Plant-Based Proteins:

Advantages: These proteins tend to have a lower purine content compared to animal-derived proteins.

Choices: Consider tofu, beans, lentils, and nuts as primary protein sources.

4. Fatty Fish:

While fatty fish like salmon, mackerel, and trout offer anti-inflammatory benefits, it's essential to consume them in moderation due to their purine content.

5. Eggs:

As a versatile protein source, eggs are a favorable choice for gout sufferers due to their lower purine content.

6. Hydration:

Significance: Keeping well-hydrated makes sure efficient uric acid flushingby the kidneys.

Guideline: While 8-10 glasses of water daily is a general recommendation, individual needs might vary.

7. Coffee:

Both caffeinated and decaffeinated coffee may offer

benefits in lowering gout risk, though the exact mechanism is still under investigation.

8. Extra-Virgin Olive Oil (EVOO):

Incorporate EVOO into the diet for its anti-inflammatory properties, which can be especially beneficial for individuals with gout.

Diving Deeper into Hydration

Hydration is not just crucial for general health but is especially significant for those with gout.

Here's why:

Efficient Uric Acid Removal:

Consuming adequate water aids the kidneys in processing and cutting uric acid, decreasing the likelihood of crystal formation in the joints.

Lowering Kidney Stone Risk:

Staying hydrated can reduce the chances of developing uric acid kidney stones.

Joint Health:

Proper hydration makes sure that joints remain lubricated, minimizing stress on them.

Supporting Metabolic Processes:

Drinking enough water supports various metabolic functions, some of which might have an indirect bearing on gout.

Assessing Hydration Levels:

General Guideline:

Around 8-10 glasses (around 2 liters or half a gallon) of water daily serves as a standard recommendation for many.

Personalized Needs:

Factors like body weight, local climate, activity levels, and overall health can infuence individual hydration requirements.

Monitoring Hydration:

A straightforward method to assess hydration is by examining urine color. A light, pale yellow indicates optimal hydration, whereas a darker hue suggests the need for increased water intake.

To wrap up, while water is fundamental in gout management, it's also vital to be cautious about other beverages, especially those rich in alcohol or sugar. For personalized guidance, especially when dealing with conditions like gout, it's always advisable to consult with a healthcare professional or nutritionist.

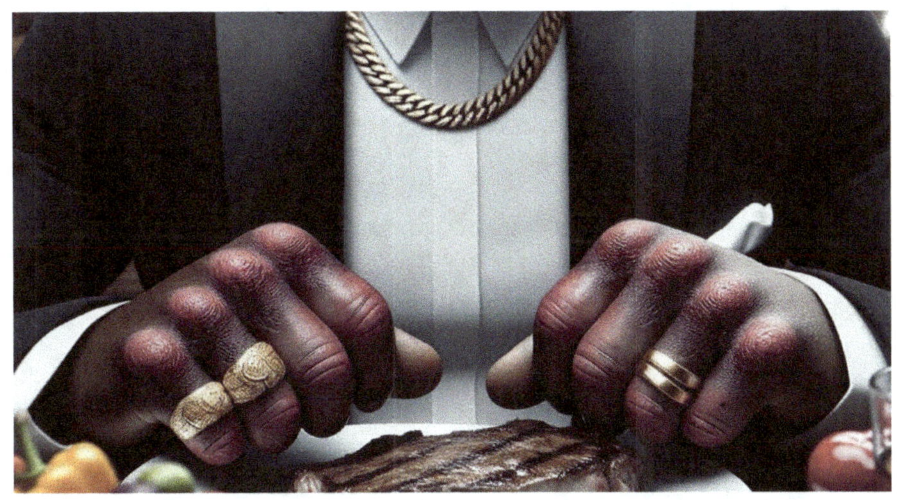

CHAPTER 8 - TREATMENT OPTIONS

Managing the symptoms of gout and preventing flare-ups is paramount for those diagnosed with the condition.

ΔΔΔ

A range of treatment options are available to address this:

Non-Steroidal Anti-Inflammatory Drugs (NSAIDs), like Ibuprofen, Naproxen, and Indomethacin, are commonly prescribed to alleviate acute pain and inflammation. Regular use, however, can result in side effects including stomach pain, heartburn, and elevated blood pressure.

Colchicine is another option, particularly during acute flare-ups or when starting a new gout medication. Notable side effects encompass nausea, diarrhea, and stomach cramps.

For patients who are unable to take NSAIDs or colchicine,

corticosteroids such as Prednisone might be recommended. While effective in controlling pain and inflammation, potential side effects include mood changes, increased blood sugar levels, and a heightened appetite.

To reduce the risk of gout attacks, Uric Acid-Lowering Medications are beneficial

Xanthine Oxidase Inhibitors, including Allopurinol and Febuxostat, decrease uric acid production. Side effects can range from rashes to nausea.
Uricosurics like Probenecid enhance uric acid elimination by the kidneys. However, they might lead to rashes, stomach pain, or kidney stones.
Uric Acid Reabsorption Inhibitors such as Lesinurad aid in uric acid removal. Some patients might experience kidney-related issues or increased blood creatinine levels.

For persistent cases resistant to standard treatments, biologics like **Pegloticase** can be considered. It aids in the breakdown of uric acid but may trigger side effects like allergic reactions or nausea.

Regardless of the chosen treatment, consulting with a healthcare professional is essential to make sure the most appropriate medication and dosage is determined, and to be aware of potential side effects.

When considering complementary therapies for gout, several natural remedies stand out:

Cherries are linked to decreased uric acid levels and fewer gout fare-ups. While generally beneficial, consuming large quantities might cause digestive discomfort. Additionally, cherries can sometimes interact with specific medications.

Apple Cider Vinegar is popular for its potential in reducing pain and inflammation. Typically, 1-2 tablespoons diluted in water are consumed daily. However, undiluted vinegar can damage tooth enamel and might have interactions with certain drugs.

Celery Seed Extract is believed to have anti-inflammatory benefits and might aid in uric acid elimination. However, it's unsuitable for certain groups, like pregnant or nursing women, and those on specific medications.

Nettle Tea functions as a diuretic, aiding in uric acid removal. Prepared by steeping nettle leaves in hot water, it might have interactions with several medications.

Dandelion is another remedy believed to be diuretic. Whether consumed as tea or supplements, those with gallbladder issues or specific medications should approach with caution.

Ginger Root is recognized for its anti-inflammatory properties. While it can be incorporated into meals, drank as tea, or applied as a topical paste, excessive intake can lead to digestive concerns and potential drug interactions.

Turmeric, containing the anti-inflammatory compound curcumin, can be used in food or taken as supplements. However, prolonged consumption or high doses might cause digestive issues and might interfere with some medications.

Bromelain, an enzyme sourced from pineapples, can alleviate gout pain due to its anti-inflammatory properties. Available as supplements, some might experience allergic reactions, and there are known drug interactions.

While these remedies can offer relief, consulting with a healthcare expert is vital to make sure they're safe to use, especially when combined with other treatments or conditions.

Lifestyle adjustments can effectively mitigate gout and decrease fare-up occurrences:

Weight Management

Purpose: Excess weight can hinder the body's uric acid removal, escalating gout attack chances.

Actions: Focus on a balanced diet with fruits, veggies, whole grains, and lean proteins. Engage in consistent exercise, blending aerobic activities and strength training.

Dietary Changes

Purpose: Some foods elevate uric acid.

Actions: Minimize high-purine foods like certain meats and seafood. Reduce alcohol and high-fructose items. Stay well-hydrated.

Limit Alcohol

Purpose: Alcohol can obstruct uric acid clearance.

Actions: Minimize alcohol, particularly beer. Wine can be a moderate alternative.

Avoid Trigger Foods

Purpose: Individual triggers can induce fare-ups.

Actions: Maintain a food diary to discern triggers and then avoid or limit them.

Stay Hydrated

Purpose: Proper hydration helps in uric acid elimination and thwarts crystal development.

Actions: Aim for 8-10 glasses of water daily and limit sugary or caffeinated drinks.

Medication Adherence

Purpose: Consistent medication intake helps control uric acid and reduces fare-up risk.

Actions: Adhere to medication guidelines and consult with your doctor for adjustments.

Regular Check-ups

Purpose: Routine checks can detect elevated uric acid before fare-ups occur.

Actions: Organize regular healthcare professional visits for uric acid monitoring and health assessment.

Stress Management

Purpose: Stress can provoke gout for some.

Actions: Embrace relaxation techniques, make sure sleep restful, and remain physically active.

Avoid Trauma

Purpose: Joint injuries can instigate gout episodes.

Actions: Exercise caution to safeguard joints, particularly previously affected ones. Wear protective gear during physical tasks or sports.

Adopting these lifestyle adaptations can enable gout sufferers to more effectively control their condition and minimize painful episodes. Collaborating with a healthcare specialist is paramount to determine the optimal gout management strategy.

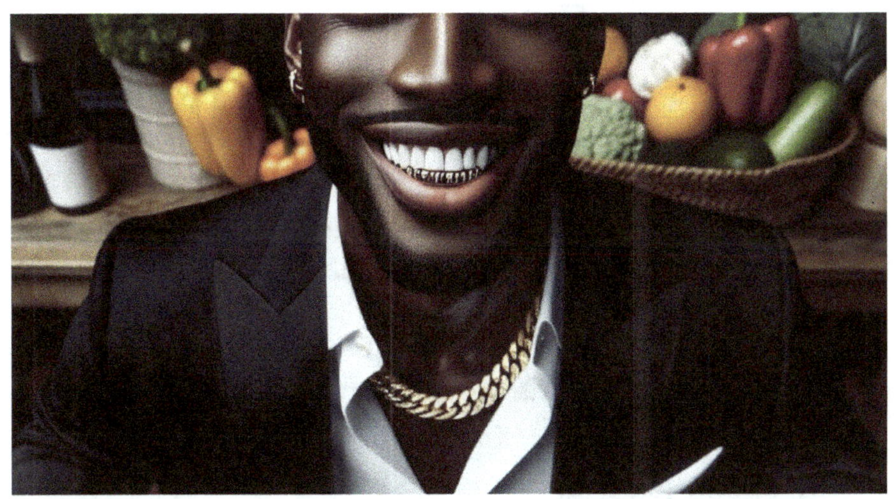

CHAPTER 9 - LIVING WITH GOUT

Living with gout can be challenging, but with the right strategies and a proactive approach, one can lead a fulfilling life while managing the condition.

ΔΔΔ

Below, we present the ABCs of effective gout management.

A. Tips for Managing Gout Pain - All hands on deck

1. Rest and Elevate:

When experiencing a gout fare-up, it's crucial to rest the affected joint and keep it elevated.

This can minimize swelling and alleviate discomfort.

2. Apply Cold Compress:

For immediate relief, apply a cold pack to the inflamed joint. This reduces inflammation and provides pain relief.

3. Over-the-Counter Pain Relievers:

Medications like ibuprofen can be helpful. However, always consult a doctor before starting any medication.

4. Stay Hydrated:

Adequate water intake aids in flushing out uric acid, thereby reducing the risk of crystal formation.

5. Wear Comfortable Shoes:

Comfortable footwear can significantly reduce pain, especially if gout affects the feet.

6. Avoid Putting Pressure on the Joint:

Keep the affected joint free from unnecessary stress, especially during a fare-up.

7. Consider Dietary Changes:

A balanced diet can both manage and prevent painful fare-ups.

8. Keep Medications on Hand:

Always be prepared. Having your prescribed gout medications ready can be a lifesaver during sudden fare-ups.

9. Maintain a Healthy Weight:

A balanced weight reduces the strain on joints, helping to minimize gout pain.

10. Manage Stress:

Since stress can be a potential trigger, consider adopting relaxation techniques.

11. Stay Informed:

Keeping abreast of the latest about gout can empower you to make the best decisions for your health.

B. The Importance of Checkups - Be proactive

1. Checking Uric Acid Levels:

Regular tests can preemptively signal a gout attack.

2. Medication Review:

Stay updated with the most effective medications tailored to your needs.

3. Diet and Lifestyle Recommendations:

As new insights emerge, stay informed through your healthcare provider.

4. Identifying Triggers:

Knowing what exacerbates your gout can significantly reduce the frequency of fare-ups.

5. Preventing Complications:

Catching potential issues early can prevent more severe complications in the future.

C.   Embracing   a   Supportive Community and Mindset

1. Join Support Groups:

Being a part of a community can provide immense emotional

support.

2. Educate Friends and Family:

The more your loved ones understand gout, the better they can support you.

3. Set Realistic Expectations:

Remember that managing gout is a journey. Celebrate progress, no matter how small.

4. Stay Updated with Research:

Knowledge is power. Stay informed about the latest in gout research.

5. Seek Mental Health Support if Needed:

Mental well-being is as crucial as physical health. Consider seeking help if you're feeling overwhelmed.

6. Practice Self-compassion:

We understand that this is a challenging condition. Be kind to yourself and acknowledge the efforts you're putting in.

Living with gout requires a blend of medical care, lifestyle adjustments, and emotional resilience. By following the ABCs outlined in this chapter, you can navigate the challenges of gout with confidence and hope. Aiming for a life with minimal pain and maximized well-being is the goal. Always remember to consult with healthcare professionals for guidance tailored to your unique needs.

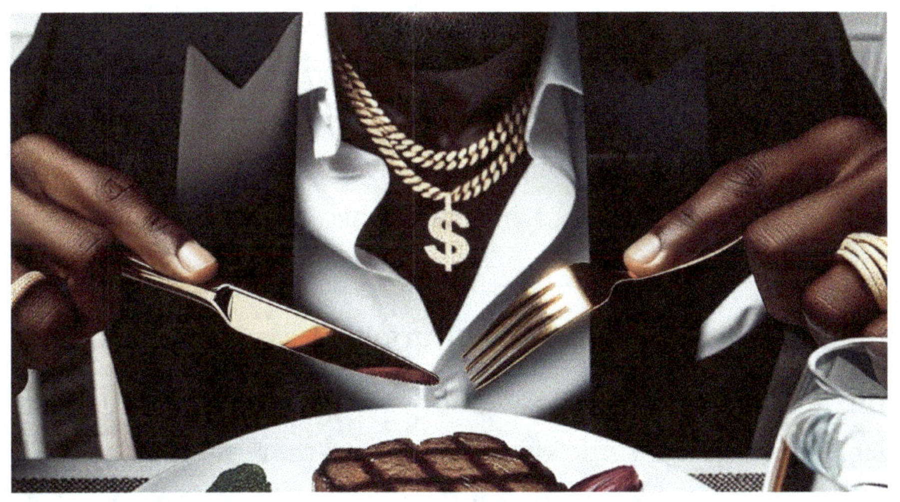

CHAPTER 10: COMMON COMORBIDITIES OF GOUT

A significant part of individuals who have been diagnosed with gout also deal with other coexisting health issues.

ΔΔΔ

This chapter delves into the most common comorbidities associated with gout, providing insight into their relationship with this condition.

1. Cardiovascular Diseases

There's a notable correlation between gout and several cardiovascular issues:

Hypertension: Around 74% of gout patients also struggle with elevated blood pressure.

Stroke & Heart Disease: Over 10% of individuals with gout experience strokes or heart-related events in their lives.

Uric acid crystals can induce inflammation within the arteries, further complicating cardiovascular matters.

2. Kidney Disease

The kidneys, pivotal in defeating uric acid, can also be affected:

Impaired Kidney Function: About 71% of gout patients exhibit signs of stage 2 chronic kidney disease or more severe stages.

This interplay between kidney functionality and gout establishes a harmful cycle where each condition exacerbates the other.

3. Obesity

Body weight plays a pivotal role in gout and its associated conditions:

Increased Risk: Higher body weight can lead to faster uric acid accumulation.

Prevalence: Roughly 53% of those diagnosed with gout also ft the obesity criteria.

Being obese can also amplify the risks for other related conditions like hypertension and diabetes.

4. Diabetes and Insulin Resistance
There's a significant overlap between gout and diabetes:

Interconnected Conditions: Research indicates that about one in four gout patients also face challenges with diabetes.

Insulin Resistance: This is when the body's cells resist insulin, calling for an increased production of this hormone.

Elevated insulin levels in gout patients can intensify the condition since insulin hinders the elimination of uric acid and sodium.

Preventative Appointments and Visits:

1. Routine Blood Tests: Essential for tracking uric acid levels and kidney health.

2. Joint X-rays: Useful for identifying damage or changes in joints.

3. Ultrasound: Helps in early detection of urate crystals in joints.

4. Dietician Consultation: Offers guidance tailored to gout-specific dietary needs.

5. Physical Therapy: Provides exercises to enhance joint health, especially post-fare-up.

Types of Doctors Specialized in Gout Management:

Rheumatologist: Expert in arthritis and related conditions.

General Practitioner (GP): Can diagnose and manage gout and facilitate coordination with specialists.

Nephrologist: Vital when there are indications of kidney issues.

Orthopedist: Beneficial if gout has caused substantial joint damage.

Dietician: Their advice can be critical in navigating gout-influenced dietary choices.

In summary, understanding the range of conditions that often go with gout equips individuals to take a comprehensive approach to their health. With consistent medical oversight and a commitment to holistic healthcare, gout's impact can be substantially reduced.

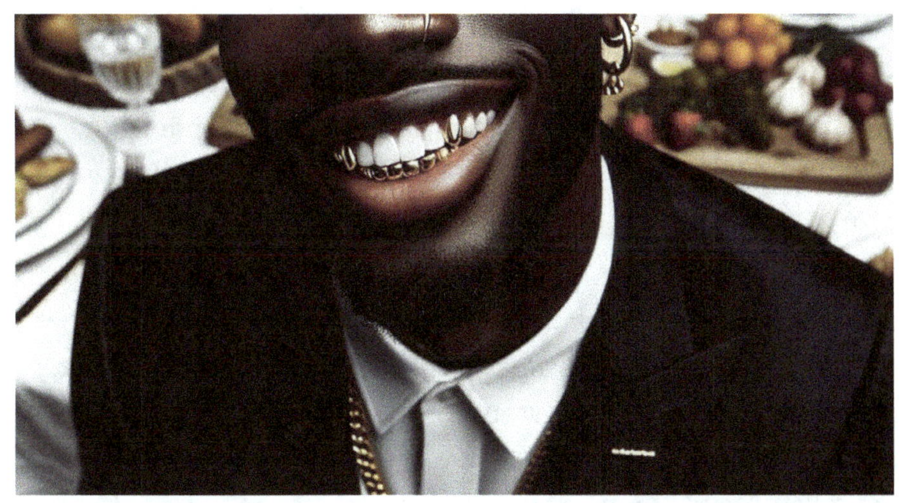

CONCLUSION – UNDERSTANDING AND MANAGING GOUT: A CRUCIAL ENDEAVOR

ΔΔΔ

Gout, often dismissed merely as a painful inconvenience, is far more than that. It's a wake-up call from our body, signaling that something is amiss. Understanding and managing gout isn't just about alleviating pain; it's about taking charge of one's overall health.

Firstly, it's essential to recognize that gout isn't an isolated issue. It intertwines with other aspects of our health, from kidney function to cardiovascular wellness. When we address gout, we're not just warding of painful fare-ups but preventing other health complications.

Moreover, understanding gout provides valuable insights into our bodies. It nudges us towards better dietary choices, underscores the importance of regular health check-ups, and teaches us the value of proactive health management. Knowledge is power, and in the realm of gout, it's the power to live pain-free and healthier.

However, managing gout isn't a solitary journey. It's a collaborative effort involving medical professionals, support groups, loved ones, and most importantly, oneself. With each step taken towards understanding and management, we move closer to a life where gout doesn't dictate our choices but merely informs them.

So, as you embark or continue on this journey of understanding and managing gout, remember:

- You're not alone. Many have walked this path and have found ways to thrive.

- Each day is a new opportunity. Every sunrise brings a chance to make healthier choices and learn more about managing gout.

- Believe in yourself. You carry the strength and resilience to tackle gout head-on and emerge even stronger.

And always remember: "You have the power to change, the strength to overcome, and the resilience to create a life you deserve." Embrace the journey, cherish the lessons, and look forward to a brighter, healthier tomorrow. You've got this! Regarding managing gout, you don't have to do it alone. Reach out to your healthcare team for support and encouragement and connect with your loved ones. Share your experiences and learn from theirs. It's okay to ask for help. There are many resources available to you, and together, you can find the best solutions for you. Leverage the support of family and friends, and don't be afraid to ask for a helping hand.

CASE STUDIES:

Introduction to Case Studies

Gout, a condition marked by intense joint pain due to the accumulation of uric acid crystals, manifests uniquely in every individual. The journey of managing, treating, and living with gout is deeply personal and varies depending on various factors including age, gender, lifestyle, and underlying health conditions.

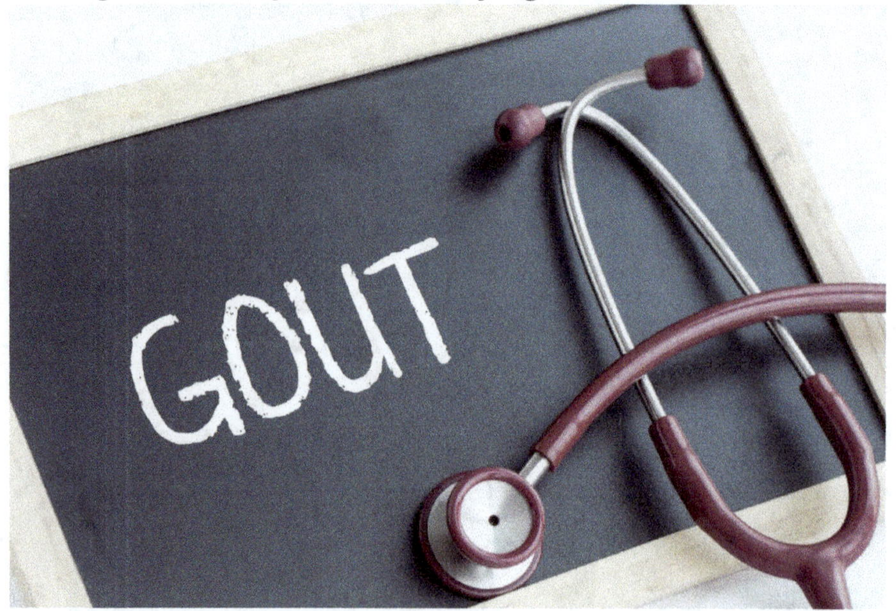

To provide a comprehensive understanding of the diverse experiences associated with gout, we present three distinct case studies.

By delving into these real-life stories, we aim to shed light on the multifaceted nature of gout and underscore the importance of personalized care, support, and understanding for those living with this condition.

ΔΔΔ

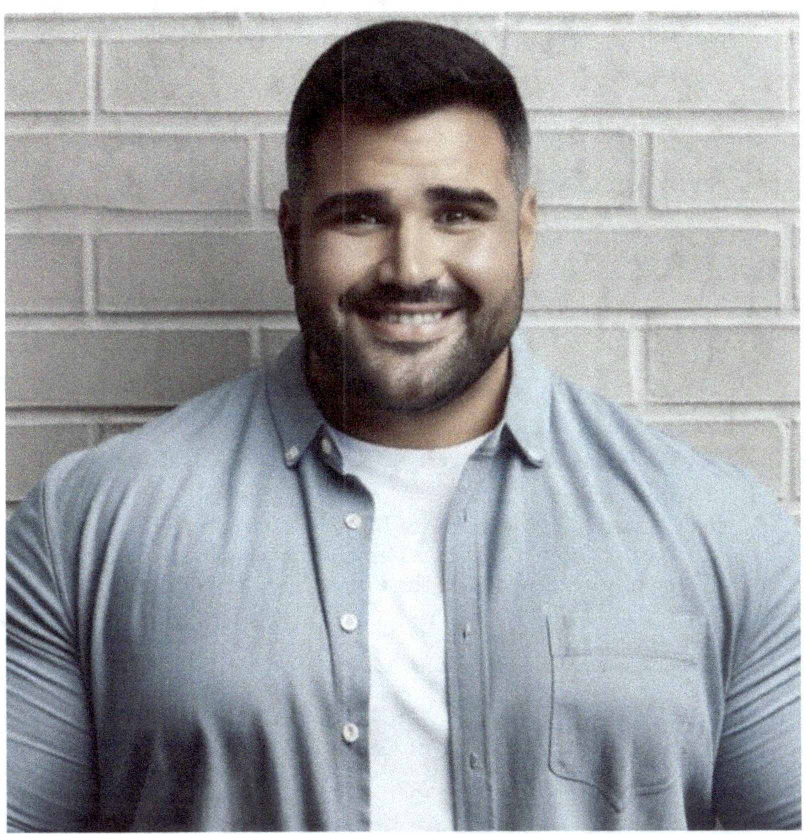

A 38-year-old male who, being in a demographic commonly affected by gout, navigates the complexities of managing the condition alongside other comorbidities and life responsibilities.

ΔΔΔ

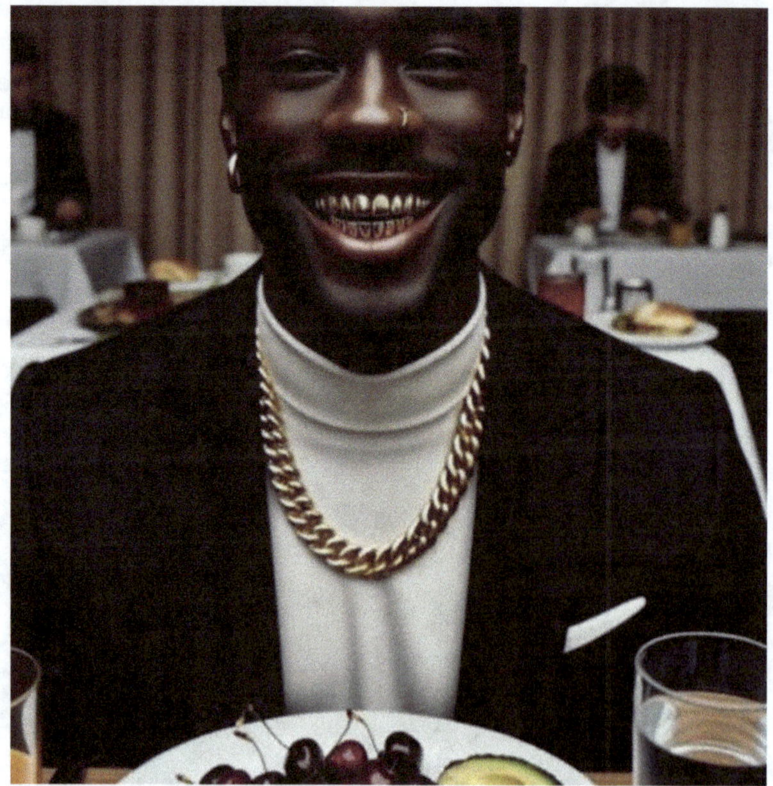

A 30-year-old man, at the prime of his life, finds himself contending with early-onset gout, offering a perspective on how the condition affects younger adults and the unique challenges they face.

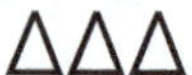

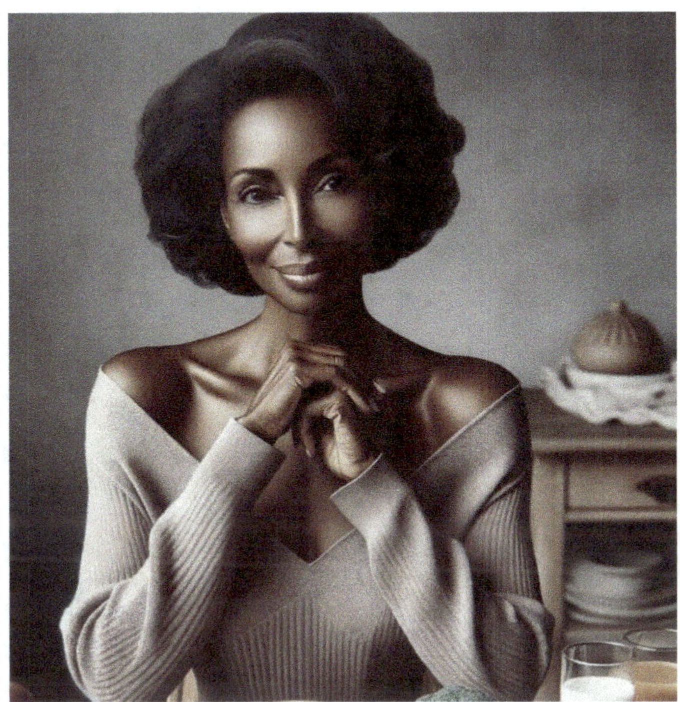

A 53-year-old woman who, despite being post-menopausal — a phase often associated with a decreased risk of gout — grapples with recurrent fare-ups and the challenge of balancing her daily routines with the unpredictability of the condition.

CASE STUDY 1: EMPOWERMENT THROUGH GOUT MANAGEMENT

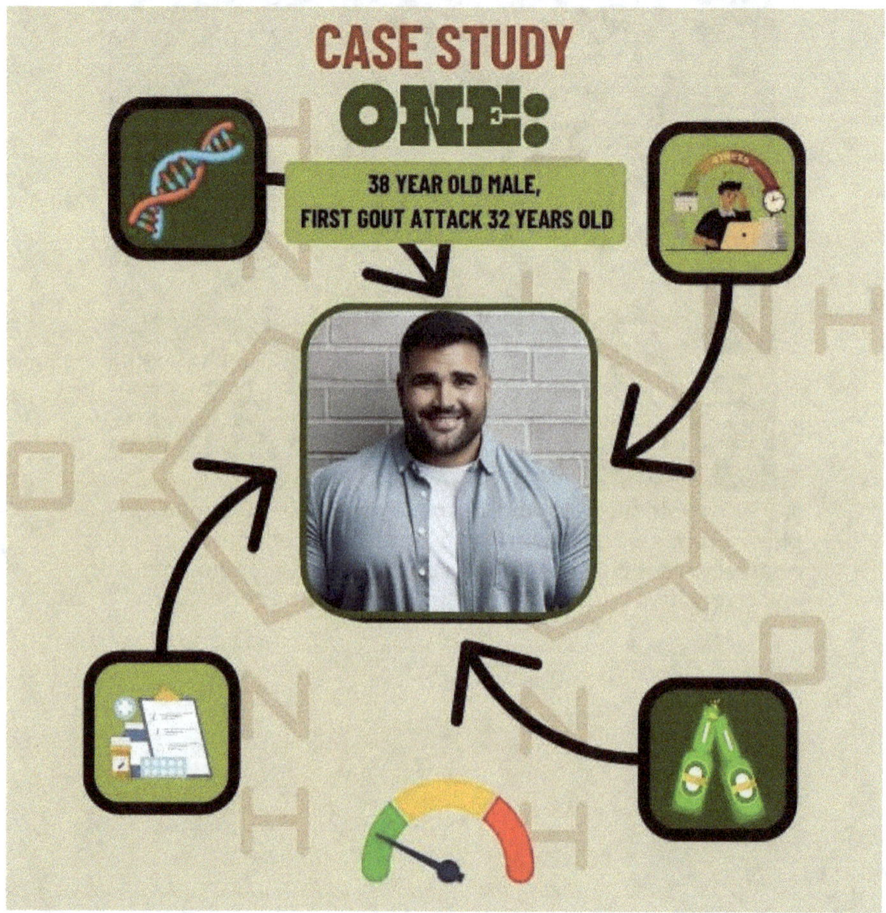

At 38, a Hispanic male with a history of bodybuilding stands tall, recalling his days of using legal steroids and growth hormones. His past as an avid beer enthusiast might have long faded, but the genetic predisposition to gout, shared by his father, grandfather, and other family members, remains a persistent challenge. Juggling the stresses of work, where the pressure is moderate, with the demands of home life is no easy feat, especially with a disabled wife and five children.

A former bodybuilder, his muscles once thrived under the influence of steroids and growth hormones. However, surgeries, like the one on his rotator cuff, hint at the toll his body has paid. Diagnosed with gout at 32, he's no stranger to the excruciating pain of its fare-ups. But gout isn't the only unwelcome guest; hypertension and chronic pain mark their presence too. Allopurinol, colchicine, and NSAIDs, alongside holistic treatments like acupuncture and anti-inflammatory herbs, make regular appearances in his battle against gout. Gout's wrath is felt in severe fare-ups, striking twice every 3-4 months. Stress, certain foods, and sometimes mysterious triggers launch these attacks. Fever, fatigue, and pain aren't just symptoms; they're constant reminders of this battle against his body.

Drawing from the Mini Playbook, he incorporates both medical and alternative treatments. A diet low in purine, with juiced low-sugar fruits and thrice-weekly alkaline foods, charts his nutritional course. Alcohol, once a favored companion, is now reserved for special occasions. Regular exercise keeps him active, a lifestyle changes as much for his gout as for himself. Monthly visits to a rheumatologist, complemented by weekly consultations with a holistic dietician, form his medical support system.

Gout casts a long shadow, dimming his social life and straining home relationships. It brings allies, too: depression and lowered immunity. But he's not one to be defeated. Physical and mental therapy sessions, coupled with acupuncture and a tailored diet, are his chosen weapons. Living with gout has taught him resilience, self-awareness, and empowerment. In his own words, "I am empowered."

His goals are clear: reduce the severity and frequency of gout attacks and reclaim his energy. Every step he takes, every choice he makes, pivots him closer to a life where gout doesn't get the final say.

CASE STUDY 2: GOUT ON THE GO

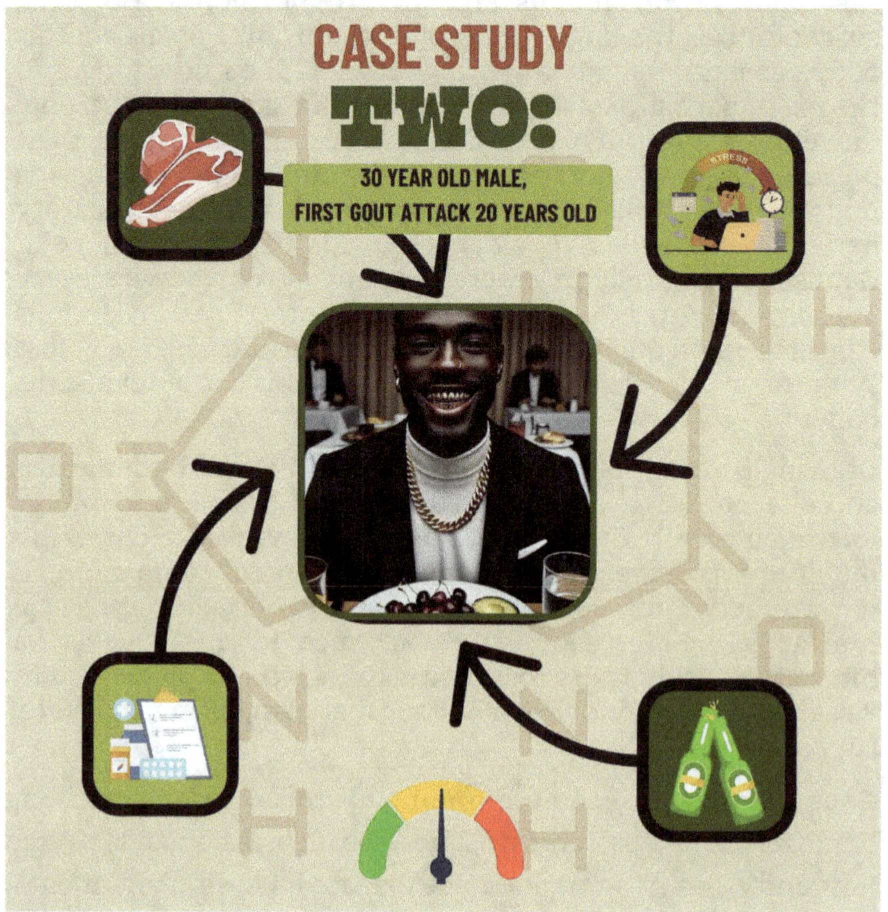

Our subject is a dedicated African American travel technician. Due to the nature of his profession, he often finds himself boarding fights, sometimes even multiple times within a single week. This constant travel, combined with the challenges of finding healthy meals while on-the-move, results in a lifestyle characterized by high stress. Beyond the immediate demands of his job, he recalls his time in the military. He reflects on certain habits from that period of his life that might have been the initial triggers for his gout.

From a medical standpoint, he first experienced a gout attack at the age of 21. Remarkably, he had no notable medical conditions before this. As of now, his only significant medical concern is gout. Over the years, he has been prescribed various treatments, including allopurinol and pain medications. Despite these prescriptions, he often finds himself deviating from the recommended treatment plan, primarily due to the side effects of these medications. This has led him to seek more natural remedies to manage his condition.

Regarding the gout experience itself, the attacks are alarmingly frequent for him. At times, the associated pain becomes almost debilitating. He identifies stress and dietary choices as the main triggers for these flare-ups. Accompanying the primary symptoms of gout are secondary issues like fatigue, irritability, and heightened pain sensations.

His approach to managing gout is multi-faceted. While he often relies on his prescribed medication, he has a marked preference for natural treatments. Dietary changes have been implemented, with red meat and pork being eliminated. He tries to make healthier food choices, although his work often challenges this initiative. When it comes to seeking professional medical advice, he tends to visit healthcare professionals based on immediate needs and availability, rather than a regular schedule.

Gout has cast a significant shadow over his personal life. There's a palpable desire in him to socialize, to be out and about. However, this is frequently sidelined by the imperative to rest and recover from gout fare-ups, leading to canceled plans and missed opportunities. Work commitments, coupled with the condition, pose significant challenges, especially when it comes to maintaining an active social life. To cope, he emphasizes stress management and ensures he gets adequate rest. Regular sessions with a therapist have also become a cornerstone of his coping mechanisms.

His journey with gout has not been without its lessons.

One profound realization he's had is the fleeting nature of life, emphasizing the importance of cherishing every moment. Looking ahead, he aspires for a life punctuated by fewer gout attacks. He hopes for increased energy levels, a healthier overall lifestyle, and more opportunities to be socially active and travel for leisure.

CASE STUDY 3: THE GARDENING GRANDMOTHER WITH GOUT

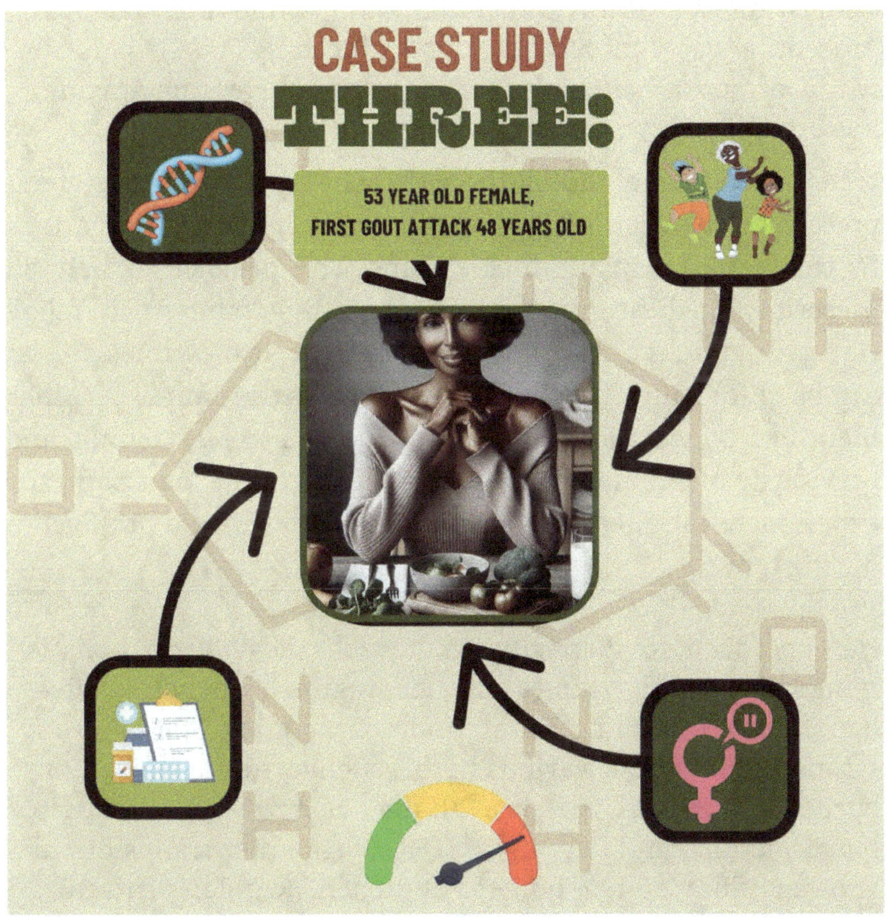

At the heart of this case is a resilient woman who gracefully juggles the roles of a mother, a grandmother, and a dedicated gardener. Having retired, she dedicates a considerable portion of her time to tending to her garden, where she cultivates fresh organic vegetables. Her commitment to a healthy lifestyle is evident in her vegan dietary choices and her daily yoga practice. While she enjoys the tranquility of her garden, her life is not without its challenges. The responsibility of caring for two of her grandchildren during the week, while her daughter serves overseas in the military, adds a significant layer of stress to her life.

Her tryst with gout began at the age of 48, an unexpected complication following an organ transplant. Notably, she underwent a kidney transplant, and while this medical procedure was vital for her, it introduced her to the painful world of gout. Menopause, another phase she's navigating, has brought its own set of challenges.

When it comes to addressing gout, she's been cautious about prescribed medications. Having linked her initial gout attack to the post-transplant medications, she decided to halt all prescribed medications, except for over-the-counter pain relief. Her gout attacks, while not very frequent at 4-6 times a year, can be quite painful, though she mentions the pain is bearable. Identified triggers for her fare-ups include stress, trauma, and previously taken medications. In addition to the joint pain, she experiences fatigue, irritability, stiffness, fever, and hot flashes during fare-ups.

Her approach to managing gout relies heavily on holistic remedies. A few staples in her regimen include coffee, lemon water, alkaline water, and cherry juice. She is also a strong proponent of various herbs, such as nettle, dandelion, burdock, horsetail, parsley, alfalfa, celery seed, turmeric, ginger, fennel, and lemongrass. Her vegan diet stands out as another pillar of her holistic approach. Regular visits to a rheumatologist, hematologist, and holistic healer/practitioner ensure she stays abreast of her health condition.

Gout, while manageable for her, occasionally becomes a hindrance. The unpredictability of attacks means there are days when she cannot engage with her grandchildren or tend to her beloved garden. To cope, she relies on stress management, ensuring she gets ample rest. She also consults a therapist, practices yoga, and uses hot/cold therapy to alleviate symptoms.

From her journey, she's derived a poignant insight: sometimes the very things we rely on for survival can harm us. Looking ahead, her aspiration is clear and simple - a life free from gout attacks.

In Conclusion: Commonalities Amid Diversity

Through these case studies, we journeyed with individuals from different walks of life, each with their unique challenges, coping mechanisms, and experiences concerning gout. While their stories were distinct, several common threads wove them together.

All three individuals identified stress as a significant trigger for their gout attacks. Whether it was the pressures of a high-paced job, caring for grandchildren, or adapting to new life phases, stress proved a ubiquitous challenge. Another shared experience was the impact of gout on their social and daily lives. Activities they loved or commitments they had were often disrupted by unpredictable fare-ups, leading to cancellations or missed opportunities.

Holistic and dietary approaches emerged as popular management strategies among the three. From vegan diets to the intake of certain beneficial foods and herbs, there was a clear inclination towards natural remedies and a cautious approach towards medication. Each individual also recognized the importance of professional medical guidance, ensuring regular check-ups with healthcare professionals relevant to their condition.

The most resonant similarity was their shared resilience. Despite the challenges, all three showcased determination in managing their condition, seeking both medical and personal ways to mitigate the effects of gout, and aspiring for a better quality of life. Their stories serve as a testament to the human spirit's capacity to adapt, learn, and thrive despite adversities.

GOUT FOOD DIARY & MOOD TRACKER

Tools for monitoring your condition more closely

Start Date: ____/____/______

Instructions:

1. Record everything you consume each day, including meals, snacks, and drinks.
2. Note the time of consumption and any immediate reactions.
3. Track any gout flare-ups or symptoms. If you experience a flare-up, try to note any potential triggers, especially foods consumed 24-48 hours prior.
4. Review this diary regularly to identify patterns or triggers.

ΔΔΔ

Week 1/Day 1:

Breakfast:
Time:________

Foods & Drinks Consumed:

1. _________________________ 2. _________________________
3. _________________________ 4. _________________________
4. _________________________ 6. _________________________

Immediate Reactions or Notes:

Lunch:
Time:_________

Foods & Drinks Consumed:

1. _________________________ 2. _________________________
3. _________________________ 4. _________________________
4. _________________________ 6. _________________________

Immediate Reactions or Notes:

Dinner:
Time:_________

Foods & Drinks Consumed:

1. _________________________ 2. _________________________
3. _________________________ 4. _________________________
4. _________________________ 6. _________________________

Immediate Reactions or Notes:

Snacks/Other:

Time:_________

Foods & Drinks Consumed:

1. _________________________ 2. _____________________________
3. _________________________ 4. _____________________________
4. _________________________ 6. _____________________________

Immediate Reactions or Notes:

GOUT FLARE-UP TRACKER:

Date: _________ Time: _________
Severity (Scale 1-10, with 10 being the most severe): _________

Affected Joints:

Potential Triggers (based on last 24-48 hours):

Symptoms Experienced:
[   ] Swelling/Inflammation
[   ] Fever
[   ] Fatigue
[   ] Other: _________________________________

____

____

Notes:

△△△

Day 2:

Breakfast:
Time:_________

Foods & Drinks Consumed:

1. _______________________ 2. _______________________
3. _______________________ 4. _______________________
4. _______________________ 6. _______________________

Immediate Reactions or Notes:

Lunch:
Time:_________

Foods & Drinks Consumed:

1. _______________________ 2. _______________________
3. _______________________ 4. _______________________
4. _______________________ 6. _______________________

Immediate Reactions or Notes:

Dinner:

Time:_________

Foods & Drinks Consumed:

1. _________________________ 2. _______________________
3. _________________________ 4. _______________________
4. _________________________ 6. _______________________

Immediate Reactions or Notes:

Snacks/Other:

Time:_________

Foods & Drinks Consumed:

1. _________________________ 2. _______________________
3. _________________________ 4. _______________________
4. _________________________ 6. _______________________

Immediate Reactions or Notes:

GOUT FLARE-UP TRACKER:

Date: _________ Time: _________
Severity (Scale 1-10, with 10 being the most severe): _________

Affected Joints:

Potential Triggers (based on last 24-48 hours):

Symptoms Experienced:
[   ] Swelling/Inflammation
[   ] Fever
[   ] Fatigue
[   ] Other: ____

____

____

Notes:

ΔΔΔ

Day 3:

Breakfast:
Time:_________

Foods & Drinks Consumed:

1. _______________________ 2. _______________________
3. _______________________ 4. _______________________
4. _______________________ 6. _______________________

Immediate Reactions or Notes:

Lunch:
Time:_________

Foods & Drinks Consumed:

1. _______________________ 2. _______________________
3. _______________________ 4. _______________________
4. _______________________ 6. _______________________

Immediate Reactions or Notes:

Dinner:
Time:_________

Foods & Drinks Consumed:

1. _______________________ 2. _______________________
3. _______________________ 4. _______________________
4. _______________________ 6. _______________________

Immediate Reactions or Notes:

Snacks/Other:
Time:_________

Foods & Drinks Consumed:

1. _________________________ 2. _____________________________
3. _________________________ 4. _____________________________
4. _________________________ 6. _____________________________

Immediate Reactions or Notes:

GOUT FLARE-UP TRACKER:

Date: _________ Time: __________
Severity (Scale 1-10, with 10 being the most severe): _________

Affected Joints:

Potential Triggers (based on last 24-48 hours):

Symptoms Experienced:
[   ] Swelling/Inflammation
[   ] Fever

[ ] Fatigue
[ ] Other: ______________________________________

____

____

Notes:

△△△

Day 4:

Breakfast:
Time:_________

Foods & Drinks Consumed:

1. ___________________ 2. ___________________
3. ___________________ 4. ___________________
4. ___________________ 6. ___________________

Immediate Reactions or Notes:

Lunch:
Time:_________

Foods & Drinks Consumed:

1. _______________________ 2. _______________________
3. _______________________ 4. _______________________
4. _______________________ 6. _______________________

Immediate Reactions or Notes:

Dinner:
Time:________

Foods & Drinks Consumed:

1. _______________________ 2. _______________________
3. _______________________ 4. _______________________
4. _______________________ 6. _______________________

Immediate Reactions or Notes:

Snacks/Other:
Time:________

Foods & Drinks Consumed:

1. _______________________ 2. _______________________
3. _______________________ 4. _______________________
4. _______________________ 6. _______________________

Immediate Reactions or Notes:

GOUT FLARE-UP TRACKER:

Date: _________ Time: _________
Severity (Scale 1-10, with 10 being the most severe): _________

Affected Joints:

Potential Triggers (based on last 24-48 hours):

Symptoms Experienced:
[   ] Swelling/Inflammation
[   ] Fever
[   ] Fatigue
[   ] Other: _________________________________

____

____

Notes:

△△△

Day 5:

Breakfast:
Time:_________

Foods & Drinks Consumed:

1. _____________________2. _______________________
3. _____________________4. _______________________
4. _____________________6. _______________________

Immediate Reactions or Notes:

Lunch:
Time:_________

Foods & Drinks Consumed:

1. _____________________2. _______________________
3. _____________________4. _______________________
4. _____________________6. _______________________

Immediate Reactions or Notes:

Dinner:
Time:_________

Foods & Drinks Consumed:

1. _____________________2. _______________________
3. _____________________4. _______________________
4. _____________________6. _______________________

Immediate Reactions or Notes:

Snacks/Other:
Time:_________

Foods & Drinks Consumed:

1. _________________________2. _________________________
3. _________________________4. _________________________
4. _________________________6. _________________________

Immediate Reactions or Notes:

GOUT FLARE-UP TRACKER:

Date: _________ Time: _________
Severity (Scale 1-10, with 10 being the most severe): _________

Affected Joints:

Potential Triggers (based on last 24-48 hours):

Symptoms Experienced:
[   ] Swelling/Inflammation
[   ] Fever

[ ] Fatigue
[ ] Other: _______________________________________

____

____

Notes:

△△△

Day 6:

Breakfast:
Time:_________

Foods & Drinks Consumed:

1. _____________________ 2. _____________________
3. _____________________ 4. _____________________
4. _____________________ 6. _____________________

Immediate Reactions or Notes:

Lunch:
Time:_________

Foods & Drinks Consumed:

1. ______________________ 2. ________________________
3. ______________________ 4. ________________________
4. ______________________ 6. ________________________

Immediate Reactions or Notes:

Dinner:

Time:________

Foods & Drinks Consumed:

1. ______________________ 2. ________________________
3. ______________________ 4. ________________________
4. ______________________ 6. ________________________

Immediate Reactions or Notes:

Snacks/Other:

Time:________

Foods & Drinks Consumed:

1. ______________________ 2. ________________________
3. ______________________ 4. ________________________
4. ______________________ 6. ________________________

Immediate Reactions or Notes:

GOUT FLARE-UP TRACKER:

Date: ___________ Time: ___________
Severity (Scale 1-10, with 10 being the most severe): ___________

Affected Joints:

Potential Triggers (based on last 24-48 hours):

Symptoms Experienced:
[   ] Swelling/Inflammation
[   ] Fever
[   ] Fatigue
[   ] Other: _______________________________________

____

____

Notes:

△△△

Day 7:

Breakfast:
Time:_________

Foods & Drinks Consumed:

1. _______________________ 2. _______________________
3. _______________________ 4. _______________________
4. _______________________ 6. _______________________

Immediate Reactions or Notes:

Lunch:
Time:_________

Foods & Drinks Consumed:

1. _______________________ 2. _______________________
3. _______________________ 4. _______________________
4. _______________________ 6. _______________________

Immediate Reactions or Notes:

Dinner:
Time:_________

Foods & Drinks Consumed:

1. _______________________ 2. _______________________
3. _______________________ 4. _______________________
4. _______________________ 6. _______________________

Immediate Reactions or Notes:

Snacks/Other:
Time:_________

Foods & Drinks Consumed:

1. _____________________2. _______________________
3. _____________________4. _______________________
4. _____________________6. _______________________

Immediate Reactions or Notes:

GOUT FLARE-UP TRACKER:

Date: _________ Time: _________
Severity (Scale 1-10, with 10 being the most severe): _________

Affected Joints:

Potential Triggers (based on last 24-48 hours):

Symptoms Experienced:
[   ] Swelling/Inflammation
[   ] Fever

[   ] Fatigue
[   ] Other: ___________________________________

____

____

Notes:

End Notes:

Oservations after week/month:

____

____

____

____

____

____

____

Common triggers identified:

____

____

____

____

____

____

Adjustments to consider for the upcoming week/month:

____
____
____
____
____
____
____

△△△

Week 2/Day 1:

Breakfast:

Time:________

Foods & Drinks Consumed:

1. ________________________ 2. ________________________
3. ________________________ 4. ________________________
4. ________________________ 6. ________________________

Immediate Reactions or Notes:

Lunch:

Time:________

Foods & Drinks Consumed:

1. ________________________ 2. ________________________
3. ________________________ 4. ________________________
4. ________________________ 6. ________________________

Immediate Reactions or Notes:

Dinner:
Time:_________

Foods & Drinks Consumed:

1. _______________________ 2. _______________________
3. _______________________ 4. _______________________
4. _______________________ 6. _______________________

Immediate Reactions or Notes:

Snacks/Other:
Time:_________

Foods & Drinks Consumed:

1. _______________________ 2. _______________________
3. _______________________ 4. _______________________
4. _______________________ 6. _______________________

Immediate Reactions or Notes:

GOUT FLARE-UP TRACKER:

Date: __________ Time: __________
Severity (Scale 1-10, with 10 being the most severe): __________

Affected Joints:

Potential Triggers (based on last 24-48 hours):

Symptoms Experienced:
[   ] Swelling/Inflammation
[   ] Fever
[   ] Fatigue
[   ] Other: _______________________________________

____

____

Notes:

△△△

Day 2:

Breakfast:
Time:__________

Foods & Drinks Consumed:

1. _______________________ 2. _______________________
3. _______________________ 4. _______________________
4. _______________________ 6. _______________________

Immediate Reactions or Notes:

Lunch:
Time:________

Foods & Drinks Consumed:

1. _______________________ 2. _______________________
3. _______________________ 4. _______________________
4. _______________________ 6. _______________________

Immediate Reactions or Notes:

Dinner:
Time:________

Foods & Drinks Consumed:

1. _______________________ 2. _______________________
3. _______________________ 4. _______________________
4. _______________________ 6. _______________________

Immediate Reactions or Notes:

Snacks/Other:
Time:_________

Foods & Drinks Consumed:

1. _______________________ 2. _______________________
3. _______________________ 4. _______________________
4. _______________________ 6. _______________________

Immediate Reactions or Notes:

GOUT FLARE-UP TRACKER:

Date: _________ Time: _________
Severity (Scale 1-10, with 10 being the most severe): _________

Affected Joints:

Potential Triggers (based on last 24-48 hours):

Symptoms Experienced:
[   ] Swelling/Inflammation
[   ] Fever
[   ] Fatigue
[   ] Other: _______________________________

____

____

Notes:

△△△

Day 3:

Breakfast:
Time:_________

Foods & Drinks Consumed:

1. _____________________ 2. _____________________
3. _____________________ 4. _____________________
4. _____________________ 6. _____________________

Immediate Reactions or Notes:

Lunch:
Time:_________

Foods & Drinks Consumed:

1. _____________________ 2. _____________________
3. _____________________ 4. _____________________

4. _____________________ 6. _____________________

Immediate Reactions or Notes:

Dinner:
Time:_________

Foods & Drinks Consumed:

1. _____________________ 2. _____________________
3. _____________________ 4. _____________________
4. _____________________ 6. _____________________

Immediate Reactions or Notes:

Snacks/Other:
Time:_________

Foods & Drinks Consumed:

1. _____________________ 2. _____________________
3. _____________________ 4. _____________________
4. _____________________ 6. _____________________

Immediate Reactions or Notes:

GOUT FLARE-UP TRACKER:

Date: _________ Time: _________
Severity (Scale 1-10, with 10 being the most severe): _________

Affected Joints:

Potential Triggers (based on last 24-48 hours):

Symptoms Experienced:
[   ] Swelling/Inflammation
[   ] Fever
[   ] Fatigue
[   ] Other: _______________________________________

____

____

Notes:

△△△

Day 4:

Breakfast:

Time:________

Foods & Drinks Consumed:

1. _________________________2. _________________________
3. _________________________4. _________________________
4. _________________________6. _________________________

Immediate Reactions or Notes:

Lunch:
Time:________

Foods & Drinks Consumed:

1. _________________________2. _________________________
3. _________________________4. _________________________
4. _________________________6. _________________________

Immediate Reactions or Notes:

Dinner:
Time:________

Foods & Drinks Consumed:

1. _________________________2. _________________________
3. _________________________4. _________________________
4. _________________________6. _________________________

Immediate Reactions or Notes:

Snacks/Other:
Time:________

Foods & Drinks Consumed:

1. ____________________ 2. ____________________
3. ____________________ 4. ____________________
4. ____________________ 6. ____________________

Immediate Reactions or Notes:

GOUT FLARE-UP TRACKER:

Date: ________ Time: ________
Severity (Scale 1-10, with 10 being the most severe): ________

Affected Joints:

Potential Triggers (based on last 24-48 hours):

Symptoms Experienced:
[ ] Swelling/Inflammation
[ ] Fever
[ ] Fatigue

[   ] Other: _______________________________________

____

____

Notes:

△△△

Day 5:

Breakfast:
Time:_________

Foods & Drinks Consumed:

1. _____________________2. _____________________
3. _____________________4. _____________________
4. _____________________6. _____________________

Immediate Reactions or Notes:

Lunch:
Time:_________

Foods & Drinks Consumed:

1. _______________________ 2. _______________________
3. _______________________ 4. _______________________
4. _______________________ 6. _______________________

Immediate Reactions or Notes:

Dinner:
Time:__________

Foods & Drinks Consumed:

1. _______________________ 2. _______________________
3. _______________________ 4. _______________________
4. _______________________ 6. _______________________

Immediate Reactions or Notes:

Snacks/Other:
Time:__________

Foods & Drinks Consumed:

1. _______________________ 2. _______________________
3. _______________________ 4. _______________________
4. _______________________ 6. _______________________

Immediate Reactions or Notes:

GOUT FLARE-UP TRACKER:

Date: _________ Time: _________
Severity (Scale 1-10, with 10 being the most severe): _________

Affected Joints:

Potential Triggers (based on last 24-48 hours):

Symptoms Experienced:
[   ] Swelling/Inflammation
[   ] Fever
[   ] Fatigue
[   ] Other: ____________________________________

____

____

Notes:

△△△

Day 6:

Breakfast:
Time:_________

Foods & Drinks Consumed:

1. _________________________ 2. _________________________
3. _________________________ 4. _________________________
4. _________________________ 6. _________________________

Immediate Reactions or Notes:

Lunch:
Time:_________

Foods & Drinks Consumed:

1. _________________________ 2. _________________________
3. _________________________ 4. _________________________
4. _________________________ 6. _________________________

Immediate Reactions or Notes:

Dinner:
Time:_________

Foods & Drinks Consumed:

1. _________________________ 2. _________________________
3. _________________________ 4. _________________________
4. _________________________ 6. _________________________

Immediate Reactions or Notes:

Snacks/Other:
Time:_________

Foods & Drinks Consumed:

1. _______________________ 2. _______________________
3. _______________________ 4. _______________________
4. _______________________ 6. _______________________

Immediate Reactions or Notes:

GOUT FLARE-UP TRACKER:

Date: _________ Time: _________
Severity (Scale 1-10, with 10 being the most severe): _________

Affected Joints:

Potential Triggers (based on last 24-48 hours):

Symptoms Experienced:
[   ] Swelling/Inflammation

[   ] Fever
[   ] Fatigue
[   ] Other: ____

____

____

Notes:

△△△

Day 7:

Breakfast:
Time:________

Foods & Drinks Consumed:

1. ________________   2. ________________
3. ________________   4. ________________
4. ________________   6. ________________

Immediate Reactions or Notes:

Lunch:
Time:________

Foods & Drinks Consumed:

1. _______________________ 2. _______________________
3. _______________________ 4. _______________________
4. _______________________ 6. _______________________

Immediate Reactions or Notes:

Dinner:
Time:________

Foods & Drinks Consumed:

1. _______________________ 2. _______________________
3. _______________________ 4. _______________________
4. _______________________ 6. _______________________

Immediate Reactions or Notes:

Snacks/Other:
Time:________

Foods & Drinks Consumed:

1. _______________________ 2. _______________________
3. _______________________ 4. _______________________
4. _______________________ 6. _______________________

Immediate Reactions or Notes:

GOUT FLARE-UP TRACKER:

Date: _________ Time: _________
Severity (Scale 1-10, with 10 being the most severe): _________

Affected Joints:

Potential Triggers (based on last 24-48 hours):

Symptoms Experienced:
[   ] Swelling/Inflammation
[   ] Fever
[   ] Fatigue
[   ] Other: ____

____

____

Notes:

End Notes:

Oservations after week/month:

____

____

____

____

____

____

Common triggers identified:

____

____

____

____

____

____

Adjustments to consider for the upcoming week/month:

____

____

____

____

____

____

△△△

Week 3/Day 1:

Breakfast:

Time:________

Foods & Drinks Consumed:

1. _________________________2. _______________________
3. _________________________4. _______________________
4. _________________________6. _______________________

Immediate Reactions or Notes:

Lunch:
Time:________

Foods & Drinks Consumed:
1. _________________________2. _______________________
3. _________________________4. _______________________
4. _________________________6. _______________________

Immediate Reactions or Notes:

Dinner:
Time:________

Foods & Drinks Consumed:

1. _________________________2. _______________________
3. _________________________4. _______________________
4. _________________________6. _______________________

Immediate Reactions or Notes:

Snacks/Other:
Time:_________

Foods & Drinks Consumed:

1. ______________________2. _______________________
3. ______________________4. _______________________
4. ______________________6. _______________________

Immediate Reactions or Notes:

GOUT FLARE-UP TRACKER:

Date: _________ Time: _________
Severity (Scale 1-10, with 10 being the most severe): _________

Affected Joints:

Potential Triggers (based on last 24-48 hours):

Symptoms Experienced:
[ ] Swelling/Inflammation
[ ] Fever

[ ] Fatigue
[ ] Other: _______________________________________

____

____

Notes:

△△△

Day 2:

Breakfast:
Time:_________

Foods & Drinks Consumed:

1. _____________________ 2. _____________________
3. _____________________ 4. _____________________
4. _____________________ 6. _____________________

Immediate Reactions or Notes:

Lunch:
Time:_________

Foods & Drinks Consumed:

1. _______________________2. _______________________
3. _______________________4. _______________________
4. _______________________6. _______________________

Immediate Reactions or Notes:

Dinner:
Time:_________

Foods & Drinks Consumed:

1. _______________________2. _______________________
3. _______________________4. _______________________
4. _______________________6. _______________________

Immediate Reactions or Notes:

Snacks/Other:
Time:_________

Foods & Drinks Consumed:

1. _______________________2. _______________________
3. _______________________4. _______________________
4. _______________________6. _______________________

Immediate Reactions or Notes:

GOUT FLARE-UP TRACKER:

Date: _________ Time: _________
Severity (Scale 1-10, with 10 being the most severe): _________

Affected Joints:

Potential Triggers (based on last 24-48 hours):

Symptoms Experienced:
[   ] Swelling/Inflammation
[   ] Fever
[   ] Fatigue
[   ] Other: _______________________________________

____

____

Notes:

ΔΔΔ

Day 3:

Breakfast:
Time:________

Foods & Drinks Consumed:

1. _________________________ 2. _____________________________
3. _________________________ 4. _____________________________
4. _________________________ 6. _____________________________

Immediate Reactions or Notes:

Lunch:
Time:________

Foods & Drinks Consumed:

1. _________________________ 2. _____________________________
3. _________________________ 4. _____________________________
4. _________________________ 6. _____________________________

Immediate Reactions or Notes:

Dinner:
Time:________

Foods & Drinks Consumed:

1. _________________________ 2. _____________________________
3. _________________________ 4. _____________________________
4. _________________________ 6. _____________________________

Immediate Reactions or Notes:

Snacks/Other:
Time:_________

Foods & Drinks Consumed:

1. _______________________ 2. _______________________
3. _______________________ 4. _______________________
4. _______________________ 6. _______________________

Immediate Reactions or Notes:

GOUT FLARE-UP TRACKER:

Date: _________ Time: _________
Severity (Scale 1-10, with 10 being the most severe): _________

Affected Joints:

Potential Triggers (based on last 24-48 hours):

Symptoms Experienced:
[ ] Swelling/Inflammation
[ ] Fever

[ ] Fatigue
[ ] Other: _______________________________________

____

____

Notes:

△△△

Day 4:

Breakfast:
Time:________

Foods & Drinks Consumed:

1. ___________________   2. ___________________
3. ___________________   4. ___________________
4. ___________________   6. ___________________

Immediate Reactions or Notes:

Lunch:
Time:________

Foods & Drinks Consumed:

1. _______________________ 2. _______________________
3. _______________________ 4. _______________________
4. _______________________ 6. _______________________

Immediate Reactions or Notes:
Dinner:
Time:_________

Foods & Drinks Consumed:

1. _______________________ 2. _______________________
3. _______________________ 4. _______________________
4. _______________________ 6. _______________________

Immediate Reactions or Notes:

Snacks/Other:
Time:_________

Foods & Drinks Consumed:

1. _______________________ 2. _______________________
3. _______________________ 4. _______________________
4. _______________________ 6. _______________________

Immediate Reactions or Notes:

GOUT FLARE-UP TRACKER:

Date: ___________ Time: ___________
Severity (Scale 1-10, with 10 being the most severe): ___________

Affected Joints:

Potential Triggers (based on last 24-48 hours):

Symptoms Experienced:
[   ] Swelling/Inflammation
[   ] Fever
[   ] Fatigue
[   ] Other: _____________________________________

____

____

Notes:

△△△

Day 5:

Breakfast:
Time:_________

Foods & Drinks Consumed:

1. ___________________________ 2. ___________________________
3. ___________________________ 4. ___________________________
4. ___________________________ 6. ___________________________

Immediate Reactions or Notes:

Lunch:
Time:_________

Foods & Drinks Consumed:

1. ___________________________ 2. ___________________________
3. ___________________________ 4. ___________________________
4. ___________________________ 6. ___________________________

Immediate Reactions or Notes:

Dinner:
Time:_________

Foods & Drinks Consumed:

1. ___________________________ 2. ___________________________
3. ___________________________ 4. ___________________________
4. ___________________________ 6. ___________________________

Immediate Reactions or Notes:

Snacks/Other:
Time:________

Foods & Drinks Consumed:

1. ______________________ 2. ______________________
3. ______________________ 4. ______________________
4. ______________________ 6. ______________________

Immediate Reactions or Notes:

GOUT FLARE-UP TRACKER:

Date: _________ Time: _________
Severity (Scale 1-10, with 10 being the most severe): _________

Affected Joints:

Potential Triggers (based on last 24-48 hours):

Symptoms Experienced:
[   ] Swelling/Inflammation

[   ] Fever
[   ] Fatigue
[   ] Other: _______________________________________

____

____

Notes:

ΔΔΔ

Day 6:

Breakfast:
Time:_________

Foods & Drinks Consumed:

1. _____________________ 2. _____________________
3. _____________________ 4. _____________________
4. _____________________ 6. _____________________

Immediate Reactions or Notes:

Lunch:
Time:_________

Foods & Drinks Consumed:

1. _________________________ 2. _________________________
3. _________________________ 4. _________________________
4. _________________________ 6. _________________________

Immediate Reactions or Notes:

Dinner:
Time:________

Foods & Drinks Consumed:

1. _________________________ 2. _________________________
3. _________________________ 4. _________________________
4. _________________________ 6. _________________________

Immediate Reactions or Notes:

Snacks/Other:
Time:________

Foods & Drinks Consumed:

1. _________________________ 2. _________________________
3. _________________________ 4. _________________________
4. _________________________ 6. _________________________

Immediate Reactions or Notes:

GOUT FLARE-UP TRACKER:

Date: _________ Time: _________
Severity (Scale 1-10, with 10 being the most severe): _________

Affected Joints:

Potential Triggers (based on last 24-48 hours):

Symptoms Experienced:
[   ] Swelling/Inflammation
[   ] Fever
[   ] Fatigue
[   ] Other: ___________________________________

____
____

Notes:

△△△

Day 7:

Breakfast:
Time:_________

Foods & Drinks Consumed:

1. _______________________ 2. _______________________
3. _______________________ 4. _______________________
4. _______________________ 6. _______________________

Immediate Reactions or Notes:

Lunch:
Time:_________

Foods & Drinks Consumed:

1. _______________________ 2. _______________________
3. _______________________ 4. _______________________
4. _______________________ 6. _______________________

Immediate Reactions or Notes:

Dinner:
Time:_________

Foods & Drinks Consumed:

1. _______________________ 2. _______________________
3. _______________________ 4. _______________________
4. _______________________ 6. _______________________

Immediate Reactions or Notes:

Snacks/Other:
Time:________

Foods & Drinks Consumed:

1. ______________________ 2. ______________________
3. ______________________ 4. ______________________
4. ______________________ 6. ______________________

Immediate Reactions or Notes:

GOUT FLARE-UP TRACKER:

Date: ________ Time: ________
Severity (Scale 1-10, with 10 being the most severe): ________

Affected Joints:

Potential Triggers (based on last 24-48 hours):

Symptoms Experienced:

[   ] Swelling/Inflammation
[   ] Fever
[   ] Fatigue
[   ] Other: _______________________________________

____

____

Notes:

End Notes:

Oservations after week/month:

____
____
____
____
____
____
____

Common triggers identified:

____
____
____
____
____
____
____

Adjustments to consider for the upcoming week/month:

____

____

____

____

____

____

____

△△△

Week 4/Day 1:

Breakfast:
Time:________

Foods & Drinks Consumed:

1. _______________________2. _______________________
3. _______________________4. _______________________
4. _______________________6. _______________________

Immediate Reactions or Notes:

Lunch:
Time:________

Foods & Drinks Consumed:

1. _______________________2. _______________________

3. _______________________ 4. _______________________
4. _______________________ 6. _______________________

Immediate Reactions or Notes:

Dinner:
Time:________

Foods & Drinks Consumed:

1. _______________________ 2. _______________________
3. _______________________ 4. _______________________
4. _______________________ 6. _______________________

Immediate Reactions or Notes:

Snacks/Other:
Time:________

Foods & Drinks Consumed:

1. _______________________ 2. _______________________
3. _______________________ 4. _______________________
4. _______________________ 6. _______________________

Immediate Reactions or Notes:

GOUT FLARE-UP TRACKER:

Date: _________ Time: _________
Severity (Scale 1-10, with 10 being the most severe): _________

Affected Joints:

Potential Triggers (based on last 24-48 hours):

Symptoms Experienced:
[   ] Swelling/Inflammation
[   ] Fever
[   ] Fatigue
[   ] Other: _______________________________________

____

____

Notes:

ΔΔΔ

Day 2:

Breakfast:

Time:________

Foods & Drinks Consumed:

1. ________________________ 2. ________________________
3. ________________________ 4. ________________________
4. ________________________ 6. ________________________

Immediate Reactions or Notes:

Lunch:
Time:________

Foods & Drinks Consumed:

1. ________________________ 2. ________________________
3. ________________________ 4. ________________________
4. ________________________ 6. ________________________

Immediate Reactions or Notes:

Dinner:
Time:________

Foods & Drinks Consumed:

1. ________________________ 2. ________________________
3. ________________________ 4. ________________________
4. ________________________ 6. ________________________

Immediate Reactions or Notes:

Snacks/Other:
Time:________

Foods & Drinks Consumed:

1. ____________________ 2. ______________________
3. ____________________ 4. ______________________
4. ____________________ 6. ______________________

Immediate Reactions or Notes:

GOUT FLARE-UP TRACKER:

Date: _________ Time: _________
Severity (Scale 1-10, with 10 being the most severe): _________

Affected Joints:

Potential Triggers (based on last 24-48 hours):

Symptoms Experienced:
[ ] Swelling/Inflammation
[ ] Fever
[ ] Fatigue

[   ] Other: _______________________________________

____

____

Notes:

△△△

Day 3:

Breakfast:
Time:__________

Foods & Drinks Consumed:

1. _____________________ 2. _____________________
3. _____________________ 4. _____________________
4. _____________________ 6. _____________________

Immediate Reactions or Notes:

Lunch:
Time:__________

Foods & Drinks Consumed:

1. _________________________ 2. _________________________
3. _________________________ 4. _________________________
4. _________________________ 6. _________________________

Immediate Reactions or Notes:

Dinner:
Time:_________

Foods & Drinks Consumed:

1. _________________________ 2. _________________________
3. _________________________ 4. _________________________
4. _________________________ 6. _________________________

Immediate Reactions or Notes:

Snacks/Other:
Time:_________

Foods & Drinks Consumed:

1. _________________________ 2. _________________________
3. _________________________ 4. _________________________
4. _________________________ 6. _________________________

Immediate Reactions or Notes:

GOUT FLARE-UP TRACKER:

Date: _________ Time: _________
Severity (Scale 1-10, with 10 being the most severe): _________

Affected Joints:

Potential Triggers (based on last 24-48 hours):

Symptoms Experienced:
[   ] Swelling/Inflammation
[   ] Fever
[   ] Fatigue
[   ] Other: ________________________________

____

____

Notes:

△△△

Day 4:

Breakfast:

Time:_________

Foods & Drinks Consumed:

1. _______________________ 2. _________________________
3. _______________________ 4. _________________________
4. _______________________ 6. _________________________

Immediate Reactions or Notes:

Lunch:
Time:_________

Foods & Drinks Consumed:

1. _______________________ 2. _________________________
3. _______________________ 4. _________________________
4. _______________________ 6. _________________________

Immediate Reactions or Notes:

Dinner:
Time:_________

Foods & Drinks Consumed:

1. _______________________ 2. _________________________
3. _______________________ 4. _________________________
4. _______________________ 6. _________________________

Immediate Reactions or Notes:

Snacks/Other:
Time:________

Foods & Drinks Consumed:

1. ___________________2. _____________________
3. ___________________4. _____________________
4. ___________________6. _____________________

Immediate Reactions or Notes:

GOUT FLARE-UP TRACKER:

Date: _________ Time: _________
Severity (Scale 1-10, with 10 being the most severe): _________

Affected Joints:

Potential Triggers (based on last 24-48 hours):

Symptoms Experienced:
[ ] Swelling/Inflammation
[ ] Fever
[ ] Fatigue

[   ] Other: _______________________________________

____

____

Notes:

△△△

Day 5:

Breakfast:
Time:_________

Foods & Drinks Consumed:

1. _____________________ 2. _____________________
3. _____________________ 4. _____________________
4. _____________________ 6. _____________________

Immediate Reactions or Notes:

Lunch:
Time:_________

Foods & Drinks Consumed:

1. _______________________ 2. _______________________
3. _______________________ 4. _______________________
4. _______________________ 6. _______________________

Immediate Reactions or Notes:

Dinner:

Time:_________

Foods & Drinks Consumed:

1. _______________________ 2. _______________________
3. _______________________ 4. _______________________
4. _______________________ 6. _______________________

Immediate Reactions or Notes:

Snacks/Other:

Time:_________

Foods & Drinks Consumed:

1. _______________________ 2. _______________________
3. _______________________ 4. _______________________
4. _______________________ 6. _______________________

Immediate Reactions or Notes:

GOUT FLARE-UP TRACKER:

Date: _________ Time: _________
Severity (Scale 1-10, with 10 being the most severe): _________

Affected Joints:

Potential Triggers (based on last 24-48 hours):

Symptoms Experienced:
[   ] Swelling/Inflammation
[   ] Fever
[   ] Fatigue
[   ] Other: ____

____

____

Notes:

ΔΔΔ

Day 6:

Breakfast:

Time:_________

Foods & Drinks Consumed:

1. _________________________ 2. _________________________
3. _________________________ 4. _________________________
4. _________________________ 6. _________________________

Immediate Reactions or Notes:

Lunch:
Time:_________

Foods & Drinks Consumed:

1. _________________________ 2. _________________________
3. _________________________ 4. _________________________
4. _________________________ 6. _________________________

Immediate Reactions or Notes:

Dinner:
Time:_________

Foods & Drinks Consumed:

1. _________________________ 2. _________________________
3. _________________________ 4. _________________________
4. _________________________ 6. _________________________

Immediate Reactions or Notes:

Snacks/Other:
Time:________

Foods & Drinks Consumed:

1. ________________________2. ________________________
3. ________________________4. ________________________
4. ________________________6. ________________________

Immediate Reactions or Notes:

GOUT FLARE-UP TRACKER:

Date: ________ Time: ________
Severity (Scale 1-10, with 10 being the most severe): ________

Affected Joints:

Potential Triggers (based on last 24-48 hours):

Symptoms Experienced:
[ ] Swelling/Inflammation
[ ] Fever
[ ] Fatigue

[   ] Other: ______________________________________

____

____

Notes:

△△△

Day 7:

Breakfast:
Time:________

Foods & Drinks Consumed:

1. ___________________ 2. ___________________
3. ___________________ 4. ___________________
4. ___________________ 6. ___________________

Immediate Reactions or Notes:

Lunch:
Time:________

Foods & Drinks Consumed:

1. _______________________ 2. _______________________
3. _______________________ 4. _______________________
4. _______________________ 6. _______________________

Immediate Reactions or Notes:

Dinner:
Time:_________

Foods & Drinks Consumed:

1. _______________________ 2. _______________________
3. _______________________ 4. _______________________
4. _______________________ 6. _______________________

Immediate Reactions or Notes:

Snacks/Other:
Time:_________

Foods & Drinks Consumed:

1. _______________________ 2. _______________________
3. _______________________ 4. _______________________
4. _______________________ 6. _______________________

Immediate Reactions or Notes:

GOUT FLARE-UP TRACKER:

Date: __________ Time: __________
Severity (Scale 1-10, with 10 being the most severe): __________

Affected Joints:

Potential Triggers (based on last 24-48 hours):

Symptoms Experienced:
[   ] Swelling/Inflammation
[   ] Fever
[   ] Fatigue
[   ] Other: ____

____

____

Notes:

End Notes:

Oservations after week/month:

Common triggers identified:

Adjustments to consider for the upcoming week/month:

Gout affects both physical health and emotional well-being. Use this Gout Mood Tracker to capture daily feelings and symptoms, helping you discern patterns and navigate your journey with deeper insight.

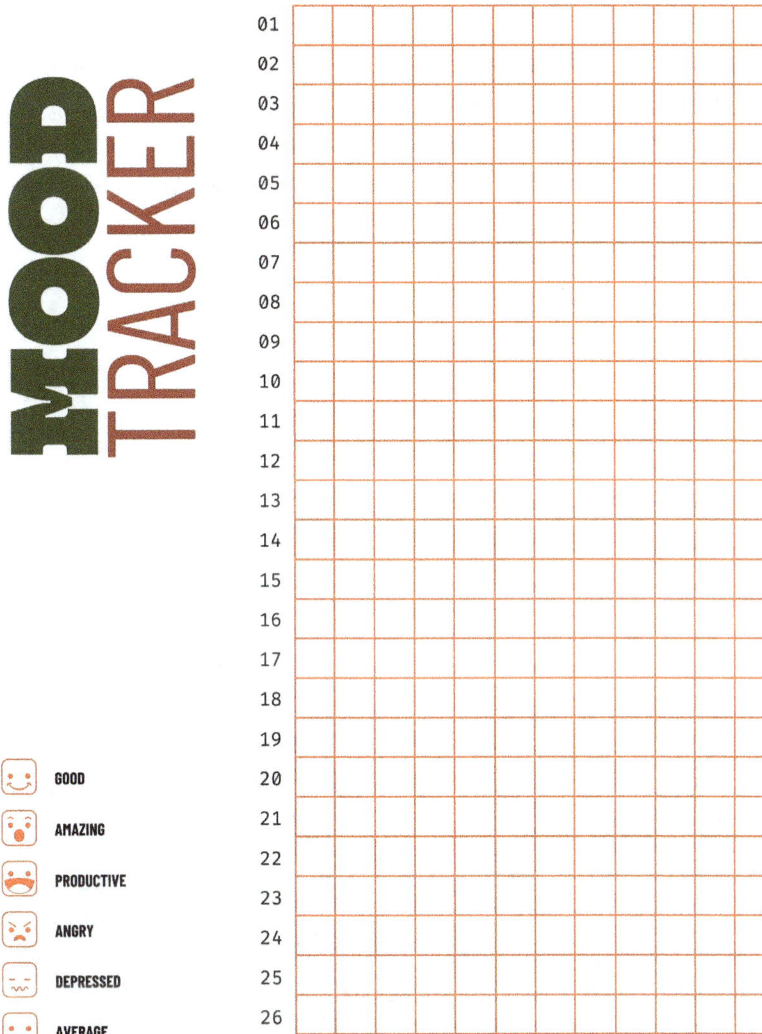

Using these tools is entirely optional, and readers are wholeheartedly encouraged to devise their own methods for monitoring their condition and mood. Remember, personalization often leads to the best understanding and management of one's well-being.

Don't forget that keeping an accurate diary will help in understanding patterns, identifying potential triggers, and making informed choices for better managing gout. Regularly review and discuss this diary with your healthcare professional.

△△△

AFTERWORD

As we close the pages on "Deeper than Gout: An Average Guide to the Rich Man's Disease," I am filled with gratitude for your willingness to accompany me on this explorative journey. Gout is far more than a mere medical condition; it's a maze of personal stories, experiences, challenges, and triumphs. Through the lens of this guide, I hope you've gained not only knowledge but also empathy for those navigating the complexities of this ailment.

While the information and stories shared in this e-book provide insight and awareness, the journey with gout doesn't end here. Practical strategies, consistent efforts, and informed choices can make a world of difference in managing and even preventing debilitating flare-ups. With that spirit in mind, I am delighted to offer you a Free Mini-Strategy Playbook. This playbook is designed to be your ally, offering actionable strategies, tips, recipes, and methods to manage gout flare-ups and enrich your quality of life.

[Click here to download your Mini-Strategy Playbook for managing gout flare-ups.]

Beyond the medical advice and prescriptions, remember that a community stands with you. Together, we share, learn, and strive for a life where gout doesn't define us, but where our resilience in the face of it does.

Thank you for being a part of this journey. I hope the insights from this e-book and the strategies from the playbook empower you to walk confidently, knowing that a life with gout can still be a life full of richness, in all senses of the word.

Warmly,
J